A Feast of Information

For people who love to eat but need to know the calorie count of their meals. This extraordinary guide lists thousands of basic and ready-to-eat foods, from appetizers to desserts, soups to main dishes. It's small and compact—carry it to the supermarket, to the restaurant, to the beach, to the coffee cart, and on trips. Mix, match, and keep track of the calories as they add up.

So whether you're enjoying a beef fajita pita at Jack in the Box or lounging around the pool sipping Mr. Boston margaritas, *Barbara Kraus 1992 Calorie Guide to Brand Names and Basic Foods* makes it easy to learn the calorie count of many of your favorite foods and drinks.

BARBARA KRAUS
1992 CALORIE GUIDE
TO BRAND NAMES
AND BASIC FOODS

Barbara Kraus 1992 Calorie Guide to Brand Names and Basic Foods

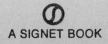

A SIGNET BOOK

For Ginna Lass

SIGNET
Published by the Penguin Group
Penguin Books USA Inc., 375 Hudson Street,
New York, New York 10014, U.S.A.
Penguin Books Ltd, 27 Wrights Lane,
London W8 5TZ, England
Penguin Books Australia Ltd, Ringwood,
Victoria, Australia
Penguin Books Canada Ltd, 10 Alcorn Avenue,
Toronto, Ontario, Canada M4V 3B2
Penguin Books (N.Z.) Ltd, 182-190 Wairau Road,
Auckland 10, New Zealand

Penguin Books Ltd, Registered Offices:
Harmondsworth, Middlesex, England

First published by Signet, an imprint of New American Library, a
division of Penguin Books USA Inc.

First Printing, January, 1992
10 9 8 7 6 5 4 3 2 1

Excerpted from *Dictionary of Calories and Carbohydrates*

 REGISTERED TRADEMARK—MARCA REGISTRADA

Printed in the United States of America

Foreword

The composition of the foods we eat is not static: it changes from time to time. In the case of *brand-name* products, manufacturers alter their recipes to reflect the availability of ingredients, advances in technology, or improvements in formulae. Each year new products appear on the market and some old ones are discontinued.

On the other hand, information on *basic foods* such as meats, vegetables, and fruits may also change as a result of the development of better analytical methods, different growing conditions, or new marketing practices. These changes, however, are usually relatively small as compared with those in manufactured products.

Some differences may be found between the values in this book and those appearing on the product labels. This is usually due to the fact that the Food and Drug Administration permits manufacturers to round the figures reported on labels. The data in this book are reported as calculated without rounding. If large differences between the two sets of values are noted, they may be due to changes in product formulae, and in those cases the label data should be used.

For all these reasons, a book of calorie or nutritive values of foods must be kept up to date by a periodic review and revision of the data presented.

Therefore, this handy calorie counter will provide each year the most current and accurate estimates available. Generous use of this little book will help you and your family to select the right foods and the proper number of calories each member requires to gain, lose, or maintain healthy and attractive weight.

Barbara Kraus

Why This Book?

Some of the data presented here can be found in more detail in my best-selling *Calories and Carbohydrates*, a dictionary of more than 8,000 brand names and basic foods. Complete as it is, it is meant to be used as a reference book at home or in the office and not to be squeezed into a suit jacket or evening bag—it's just too big.

Therefore, responding to the need for a portable calorie guide, and one which can reflect food changes often, I have written this smaller and handier version. The selection of material and the additional new entries provide readers with pertinent data on thousands of products that they would prepare at home to take to work, eat in a restaurant or luncheonette, nibble on from the coffee cart, take to the beach, buy in the candy store, et cetera.

For the sake of saving space and providing you with a greater selection of products, I had to make certain compromises: whereas in the giant book there are several physical descriptions of a product, here there is but one.

For Beginners Only

The language of dieting is no more difficult to learn than any other new subject; in many respects, it's much easier, particularly if you restrict your education to clearly defined goals.

For you who never before had the need or the interest in a lesson in weight control, I offer the following elementary introduction, applicable to any diet, self-initiated or suggested by your doctor, nutritionist, or dietician.

A Calorie

An analysis of foods in terms of calories is most often the chosen method to describe the relative energy yielded by foods.

A calorie is a shorthand way to summarize the units of energy contained in any foodstuff or alcoholic beverage, similar to the way a thermometer indicates heat. One pound of fat is equal to 3,500 calories. Add this number of calories to those you need to balance your energy requirements and you will gain one pound; subtract it and you will lose a pound.

Other Nutrients

Carbohydrates—which include sugars, starches, and acids—are only one of several chemical compounds in foods that yield calories. Proteins, found mainly in beef, poultry, and fish; fats, found in oils, butter, marbling of meat, and poultry skin; and alcohol, found in some beverages, also contribute calories. Except for alcohol, most foods contain at least some of these nutrients.

The amount of carbohydrates varies from zero in meats and a trace in alcohol to a heavy concentration in sugar, syrups, some fruits, grains, and root vegetables.

As of this date, the most respected nutritional researchers insist that some carbohydrates are necessary every day for maintaining good health. The amount to be included is an individual matter, and in any drastic effort to change your eating patterns, be sure to consult your doctor first.

Now, on how to use this new language.

To begin with, you use this book like a dictionary. If your plan is to cut down on calories, the easiest way to do so is to consult the portable calorie counter and keep an accurate count of your total intake of food and beverages for a period of seven days. If you have not gained or lost weight during that week, divide that number by seven and you'll have your maintenance diet expressed in calories. To lose weight, you must reduce your daily or weekly intake of calories below this maintenance level. (To gain, increase the intake.)

Keeping in mind that you want to stay healthy and eat well-balanced meals (which include the basic food groups: milk or milk products; meat, poultry, or fish; vegetables and fruits; and whole grain or enriched breads or cereals, as well as some fats or oils), you then start to cut down on your portion in order to reduce your intake of calories. There are many imaginative ways to diet without total withdrawal from one's favorite foods.

Once you know and don't have to guess what calories are in your foods, you can relax and enjoy them. It could turn out that dieting isn't so bad after all.

ABBREVIATIONS AND SYMBOLS

* = prepared as package directs[1]
< = less than
& = and
" = inch
canned = bottles or jars as well as cans
dia. = diameter
fl. = fluid
liq. = liquid
lb. = pound
med. = medium

oz. = ounce
pkg. = package
pt. = pint
qt. = quart
T. = tablespoon
Tr. = trace
sq. = square
tsp. = teaspoon
wt. = weight

Italics or name in parentheses = registered trademark, ®. All data not identified by company or trademark are based on material obtained from the United States Department of Agriculture or Health and Human Services (formerly Health, Education and Welfare)/Food and Agriculture Organization.

EQUIVALENTS

By Weight
1 pound = 16 ounces
1 ounce = 28.35 grams
3.52 ounces = 100 grams

By Volume
1 quart = 4 cups
1 cup = 8 fluid ounces
1 cup = ½ pint
1 cup = 16 tablespoons
2 tablespoons = 1 fluid ounce
1 tablespoon = 3 teaspoons
1 pound butter = 4 sticks or 2 cups

[1]If the package directions call for whole or skim milk, the data given here are for whole milk unless otherwise stated.

A

Food and Description	Measure or Quantity	Calories
ABALONE, canned	4 oz.	91
AC'CENT	¼ tsp.	3
AGNELOTTI, frozen (Buitoni):		
Cheese filled	2-oz. serving	196
Meat filled	2-oz. serving	206
ALBACORE, raw, meat only	4 oz.	201
ALLSPICE (French's)	1 tsp.	6
ALMOND:		
In shell	10 nuts	60
Shelled, raw, natural, with skins	1 oz.	170
Roasted, dry (Planters)	1 oz.	170
Roasted, honey (Eagle)	1 oz.	150
Roasted, oil (Tom's)	1 oz.	180
ALMOND BUTTER (Hain):		
Raw, natural	1 T.	95
Toasted, blanched	1 T.	105
ALMOND DELIGHT, cereal (Ralston Purina)	¾ cup (1 oz.)	110
ALMOND EXTRACT, pure (Durkee)	1 tsp.	13
ALPHA-BITS, cereal (Post)	1 cup (1 oz.)	110
AMARETTO DI SARONNO	1 fl. oz.	83
ANCHOVY, PICKLED, canned, flat or rolled, not heavily salted, drained (Granadaisa)	2-oz. can	80
ANISE EXTRACT, imitation (Durkee)	1 tsp.	16
ANISETTE:		
(DeKuyper)	1 fl. oz.	95
(Mr. Boston)	1 fl. oz.	88
APPLE:		
Fresh, with skin	2½″ dia.	61
Fresh, without skin	2½″ dia.	53
Canned:		
(Comstock):		
Rings, drained	1 ring	30
Sliced	⅙ of 21-oz. can	45
(White House):		
Rings	1 ring	11
Sliced	½ cup (4 oz.)	54

1

Food and Description	Measure or Quantity	Calories
Dried:		
(Del Monte)	1 cup	140
(Sun-Maid/Sunsweet)	2-oz. serving	150
(Weight Watchers):		
Chips	¾-oz. pouch	70
Snack	.5-oz. pouch	50
Frozen, sweetened	1 cup	325
APPLE BROWN BETTY	1 cup	325
APPLE BUTTER:		
(Bama)	1 T.	36
(Home Brands)	1 T.	52
(Smucker's)	1 T.	38
(White House)	1 T.	38
APPLE CHERRY BERRY DRINK, canned (Lincoln)	6 fl. oz.	90
APPLE CHERRY JUICE, canned (Red Cheek)	6 fl. oz.	113
APPLE CIDER:		
Canned:		
(Johanna Farms)	½ cup	56
(Tree Top)	6 fl. oz.	90
*Frozen (Tree Top)	6 fl. oz.	90
*Mix, *Country Time*	8 fl. oz.	98
APPLE CITRUS JUICE (Tree Top), canned or *frozen	6 fl. oz.	90
APPLE-CRANBERRY JUICE, canned (Lincoln)	6 fl. oz.	100
APPLE DRINK, canned:		
Capri Sun, natural	6¾ fl. oz.	90
Ssips (Johanna Farms)	8.45-fl.-oz. container	130
APPLE DUMPLINGS, frozen (Pepperidge Farm)	1 dumpling	260
APPLE, ESCALLOPED:		
Canned (White House)	½ cup (4.5 oz.)	163
Frozen (Stouffer's)	4 oz.	130
APPLE-GRAPE JUICE:		
Canned:		
(Mott's)	8.45-fl.-oz. container	128
(Red Cheek)	6 fl. oz.	109
(Tree Top)	6 fl. oz.	100
*Frozen (Tree Top)	6 fl. oz.	100
APPLE JACKS, cereal (Kellogg's)	1 cup (1 oz.)	110
APPLE JAM (Smucker's)	1 T.	53
APPLE JELLY:		
Sweetened:		
(Bama)	1 T.	45
(Home Brands)	1 T.	52
(Smucker's)	1 T.	54
Dietetic:		

Food and Description	Measure or Quantity	Calories
(Estee; Featherweight; Louis Sherry)	1 T.	6
(Diet Delight)	1 T.	12
APPLE JUICE:		
Canned:		
(Borden) *Sippin' Pak*	8.45-fl.-oz. container	110
(Johanna Farms) *Tree Ripe*	8.45-fl.-oz. container	121
(Land O'Lakes)	6 fl. oz.	90
(Libby's)	6 fl. oz.	78
(Lincoln) cocktail	6 fl. oz.	90
(Minute Maid)	6 fl. oz.	100
(Mott's)	6 fl. oz.	88
(Ocean Spray)	6 fl. oz.	90
(Red Cheek)	6 fl. oz.	85
(Tree Top) regular	6 fl. oz.	90
(White House)	6 fl. oz.	87
Chilled (Minute Maid)	6 fl. oz.	91
*Frozen:		
(Minute Maid)	6 fl. oz.	91
(Sunkist)	6 fl. oz.	59
(Tree Top)	6 fl. oz.	90
APPLE JUICE DRINK, canned:		
Squeezit (General Mills)	6¾-oz. bottle	110
(Sunkist)	8.5 fl. oz.	140
APPLE NECTAR, canned (Libby's)	6 fl. oz.	100
APPLE PEAR JUICE, canned or		
*frozen (Tree Top)	6 fl. oz.	90
APPLE PIE (See PIE, Apple)		
APPLE RAISIN CRISP, cereal		
(Kellogg's)	⅔ cup	130
APPLE RASPBERRY DRINK,		
canned (Mott's)	10-fl.-oz. container	158
APPLE RASPBERRY JUICE:		
Canned, regular pack:		
(Mott's)	8.45-fl.-oz. container	124
(Red Cheek)	6 fl. oz.	113
(Tree Top)	6 fl. oz.	80
*Frozen (Tree Top)	6 fl. oz.	80
APPLE SAUCE:		
Regular:		
(Hunt's) *Snack Pak:*		
Regular	4¼ oz.	50
Raspberry	4¼ oz.	80
(Mott's):		
Regular, jarred:		
Regular	6 oz.	150
Cinnamon	6 oz.	152
Single-serve cups:		
Regular	4 oz.	100

3

Food and Description	Measure or Quantity	Calories
Cherry	3¾ oz.	72
Peach	3¾ oz.	75
Strawberry	3¾ oz.	76
(Tree Top) original	½ cup	80
(White House) regular or chunky	½ cup	80
Dietetic:		
(Del Monte, lite; Diet Delight)	½ cup	50
(Mott's) single-serve cups	4 oz.	53
(S&W) *Nutradiet*, white or blue label	½ cup	55
(Thank You Brand)	½ cup	54
(White House)	½ cup	50
APPLE STRUDEL, frozen (Pepperidge Farm)	3 oz.	240
APRICOT:		
Fresh, whole	1 apricot	18
Canned, regular pack:		
(Del Monte) whole, or halves, peeled	½ cup	200
(Stokely-Van Camp)	1 cup	220
Canned, dietetic, solids & liq.:		
(Del Monte) Lite	½ cup	64
(Diet Delight):		
Juice pack	½ cup	60
Water pack	½ cup	35
(Featherweight):		
Juice pack	½ cup	50
Water pack	½ cup	35
(Libby's) Lite	½ cup	60
(S&W) *Nutradiet:*		
Halves, white or blue label	½ cup	50
Whole, juice	½ cup	40
Dried:		
(Del Monte; Sun-Maid; Sunsweet)	2 oz.	140
APRICOT LIQUEUR (DeKuyper)	1 fl. oz.	82
APRICOT NECTAR:		
(Ardmore Farms)	6 oz.	94
(Libby's)	6 fl. oz.	110
APRICOT PRESERVE:		
Sweetened (Home Brands)	1 T.	51
Dietetic (Estee)	1 T.	6
APRICOT-PINEAPPLE NECTAR, canned, dietetic (S&W) *Nutradiet*, blue label	6 oz.	35
APRICOT & PINEAPPLE PRESERVE OR JAM:		
Sweetened:		
(Home Brands)	1 T.	52
(Smucker's)	1 T.	53

Food and Description	Measure or Quantity	Calories
Dietetic:		
(Diet Delight; Louis Sherry)	1 T.	6
(S&W) *Nutradiet*	1 T.	12
ARBY'S RESTAURANT:		
Bac'n Cheddar Deluxe	1 sandwich	561
Beef & Cheddar Sandwich	1 sandwich	490
Chicken breast sandwich	7¼-oz. sandwich	592
Croissant:		
Bacon & egg	1 croissant	420
Butter	1 croissant	220
Chicken salad	1 croissant	460
Ham & swiss	1 croissant	330
Mushroom & swiss	1 croissant	340
Sausage & egg	1 croissant	530
French fries	1½-oz. serving	211
Ham 'N Cheese	1 sandwich	353
Potato cakes	2 pieces	201
Potato, stuffed:		
Broccoli & cheddar	1 potato	541
Deluxe	1 potato	648
Mushroom & cheese	1 potato	506
Taco	1 potato	619
Roast beef:		
Regular	5 oz.	353
Junior	3 oz.	218
King	6.7 oz.	467
Super	9¼ oz.	501
Garden salad (no dressing)	1 serving	165
Chef's salad (no dressing)	1 serving	235
Cashew chicken salad (contains dressing)	1 serving	505
Crackers	1 packet	25
Croutons	1 packet	70
Dressings:		
Blue cheese	1 packet	390
Buttermilk	1 packet	460
Honey French	1 packet	350
Light Italian	1 packet	25
ARTICHOKE:		
Boiled	15-oz. artichoke	187
Canned (Cara Mia) marinated, drained	6-oz. jar	175
Frozen (Birds Eye) deluxe	3 oz.	33
ASPARAGUS:		
Boiled	1 spear (½″ dia. at base)	3
Canned, regular pack, solid & liq.: (Del Monte) spears, green or white	½ cup	20

Food and Description	Measure or Quantity	Calories
(Green Giant)	½ cup	20
Canned, dietetic, solids & liq.:		
(Diet Delight)	½ cup	16
(Featherweight) cut spears	1 cup	40
(S&W) *Nutradiet*	1 cup	40
Frozen:		
(Birds Eye):		
Cuts	⅓ pkg.	22
Spears	⅓ pkg.	23
(Frosty Acres)	3.3 oz.	25
(McKenzie)	⅓ pkg.	25
(Stouffer's) souffle	⅓ pkg.	115
ASPARAGUS PILAF, frozen (Green Giant) microwave Garden Gourmet	9½-oz. pkg.	190
ASPARAGUS PUREE, canned (Larsen)	½ cup	22
AUNT JEMIMA SYRUP (See SYRUP)		
AVOCADO (Calavo)	½ fruit, edible portion (3.05 oz.)	155
AVOCADO PUREE (Calavo)	½ cup (8.1 oz.)	411
***AWAKE* (Birds Eye)**	6 fl. oz.	84

B

Food and Description	Measure or Quantity	Calories
BACON, broiled:		
(Hormel) *Black Label*	1 slice	30
(Oscar Mayer):		
Regular slice	6-gram slice	35
Center cut	1 slice	25
Thick slice	1 slice	64
BACON, CANADIAN, unheated:		
(Eckrich)	1 oz.	35
(Hormel):		
Regular	1 slice	45
Light & Lean	1 slice	17
(Oscar Mayer) 93% fat free:		
Thin	.7-oz. slice	30
Thick	1-oz. slice	35
BACON, SIMULATED, cooked:		
(Oscar Mayer) *Lean'N Tasty*:		
Beef	1 strip	48
Pork	1 strip	54
(Swift's) *Sizzlean*, pork	1 strip	35
BACON BITS:		
Bac*Os (Betty Crocker)	1 tsp.	12
(French's) imitation	1 tsp.	6
(Hormel)	1 tsp.	10
(Libby's) crumbles	1 tsp.	8
(Oscar Mayer) real	1 tsp.	6
BAGEL (Lender's):		
Plain:		
Regular	1 bagel	150
Bagelette	1 bagel	70
Egg	1 bagel	150
Onion	1 bagel	160
Poppy seed	1 bagel	160
Raisin & honey	1 bagel	200
BAKING POWDER:		
(Calumet)	1 tsp.	2
(Davis)	1 tsp.	7
(Featherweight) low sodium, cereal free	1 tsp.	8

Food and Description	Measure or Quantity	Calories
BAMBOO SHOOTS:		
Raw, trimmed	4 oz.	31
Canned, drained (Chun King)	½ cup	32
BANANA, raw (Dole)	6.3-oz. banana (weighed unpeeled)	101
BANANA EXTRACT, imitation (Durkee)	1 tsp.	15
BANANA NECTAR (Libby's)	6 fl. oz.	110
BANANA PIE (See PIE, Banana)		
BARBECUE SEASONING (French's)	1 tsp.	6
BARBERA WINE (Louis M. Martini) 12½% alcohol	3 fl. oz.	60
BARLEY, pearled (Quaker Scotch)	¼ cup	172
BASIL (French's)	1 tsp.	3
BASS:		
Baked, stuffed	3½" × 4½" × 1½"	531
Oven-fried	8¾" × 4½" × ⅝"	392
BATMAN, cereal (Ralston Purina)	1 cup	110
BAY LEAF (French's)	1 tsp.	5
B & B LIQUEUR	1 fl. oz.	94
B.B.Q. SAUCE & BEEF, frozen (Banquet) *Cookin' Bag,* sliced	4-oz. serving	100
BEAN, BAKED:		
(USDA):		
With pork & molasses sauce	1 cup	382
With pork & tomato sauce	1 cup	311
Canned:		
(Allens) *Wagon Master*	1 cup	260
(B&M) *Brick Oven:*		
Pea bean with pork in brown sugar sauce	8 oz.	300
Red kidney bean in brown sugar sauce	8 oz.	290
Vegetarian	8 oz.	250
(Campbell):		
Home style	8-oz. can	270
With pork & tomato sauce	8-oz. can	240
(Friend's):		
Pea	9-oz. serving	360
Yellow eye	9-oz. serving	360
(Furman's) & pork, in tomato sauce	8 oz.	245
(Grandma Brown's)	8 oz.	289
(Hormel) *Short Orders,* with bacon	7½-oz. can	330
(Hunt's) & pork	8 oz.	280

8

Food and Description	Measure or Quantity	Calories
BEAN, BARBECUE		
(Campbell)	7⅞-oz. can	678
BEAN & BEEF BURRITO DINNER,		
frozen (Swanson)	15¼-oz. dinner	720
BEAN, BLACK OR BROWN:		
Dry	1 cup	678
Canned:		
(Goya)	½ cup	125
(Progresso)	½ cup	90
BEAN, CHILI, canned (Hunt's)	½ cup	90
BEAN, FAVA, canned (Progresso)	4 oz.	90
BEAN & FRANKFURTER, canned:		
(Campbell) in tomato and molasses sauce	7⅞-oz. can	360
(Hormel) *Short Orders,* 'n wieners	7½-oz. can	280
BEAN & FRANKFURTER DINNER, frozen:		
(Banquet)	10-oz. dinner	520
(Morton)	10-oz. dinner	350
(Swanson)	12½-oz. dinner	550
BEAN, GARBANZO, canned:		
Regular (Old El Paso)	½ cup	190
Dietetic (S&W) *Nutradiet,* low sodium, green label	½ cup	105
BEAN, GREEN:		
Boiled, 1½″ to 2″ pieces, drained	½ cup	17
Canned, regular pack, solids & liq.:		
(Allen's):		
Whole	½ cup	21
With dry shelled beans	½ cup	40
(Del Monte)	4 oz.	20
(Green Giant) french or whole	½ cup	20
(Larsen) *Freshlike*	½ cup	20
Canned, dietetic, solids & liq.:		
(Del Monte) No Salt Added	4 oz.	19
(Diet Delight; S&W, *Nutradiet*)	½ cup	20
(Larsen) *Fresh-Lite*	½ cup	20
Frozen:		
(Birds Eye):		
Cut or french	⅓ pkg.	25
French, with almonds	3 oz.	52
Whole, deluxe	3 oz.	23
(Frosty Acres)	3 oz.	30
(Green Giant):		
Cut or french, with butter sauce, regular	3 oz.	30
Cut, *Harvest Fresh*	⅓ of 8-oz. pkg.	16
(Larsen)	3 oz.	25
(Seabrook Farms; Southland)	⅓ of 9-oz. pkg.	29

Food and Description	Measure or Quantity	Calories
BEAN, GREEN & MUSHROOM CASSEROLE (Stouffer's)	½ of 9½-oz. pkg.	160
BEAN, GREEN, WITH POTATOES, canned (Sunshine) solids & liq.	½ cup	34
BEAN, ITALIAN:		
Canned (Del Monte) solids & liq.	4 oz.	25
Frozen:		
(Birds Eye)	3 oz.	31
(Frosty Acres; Larsen)	3 oz.	30
BEAN, KIDNEY:		
Canned, regular pack, solids & liq.:		
(Allen's) red	½ cup	110
(Furman) red, fancy, light	½ cup	121
(Goya):		
Red	½ cup	115
White	½ cup	100
(Hunt's):		
Regular	4 oz.	100
Small, red	½ cup (3.5 oz.)	90
(Progresso)	½ cup	100
Canned, dietetic (S&W) *Nutradiet,* low sodium,	½ cup	90
BEAN, LIMA:		
Boiled, drained	½ cup	94
Canned, regular pack, solids & liq.:		
(Allen's):		
Regular	½ cup	60
Baby butter	½ cup	55
(Del Monte)	4 oz.	70
(Furman's)	½ cup	92
(Larsen) *Freshlike*	½ cup	80
(Sultana) butter bean	¼ of 15-oz. can	82
Canned, dietetic (Featherweight)	½ cup	80
Frozen:		
(Birds Eye) baby	⅓ pkg.	126
(Frosty Acres):		
Baby	3.3 oz.	130
Butter	3.2 oz.	140
Fordhook	3.3 oz.	100
(Green Giant):		
In butter sauce	3.3 oz	83
Harvest Fresh	3 oz.	60
(Larsen) baby	3.3 oz.	130
(Seabrook Farms):		
Baby lima	⅓ of 10-oz. pkg.	126
Baby butter bean	⅓ of 10-oz. pkg.	139
Fordhook	⅓ of 10-oz. pkg.	98

Food and Description	Measure or Quantity	Calories
BEAN, MEXICAN, canned		
(Old El Paso)	½ cup	163
BEAN, PINK, canned		
(Goya)	½ cup	115
BEAN, PINTO:		
Canned, regular pack, solids & liq.:		
(Gebhardt)	⅓ of 15-oz. can	245
(Goya) regular	½ cup (4 oz.)	100
(Green Giant)	½ cup	100
(Old El Paso)	½ cup	100
(Progresso)	½ cup	110
Frozen (McKenzie)	3.2-oz. serving	160
BEAN, RED, canned		
(Goya)	½ cup	79
BEAN, REFRIED, canned:		
(Gebhardt) regular	4 oz.	130
Little Pancho, & green chili	½ cup	80
(Old El Paso):		
Plain	½ cup	110
With bacon	½ cup	208
With green chilis	½ cup	98
With sausage	½ cup	360
Vegetarian	½ cup	140
(Rosarita):		
Regular	4 oz.	130
With green chilis	4 oz.	116
Spicy	½ cup	120
Vegetarian	½ cup	120
BEAN, ROMAN, canned:		
(Goya)	½ cup	81
(Progresso)	½ cup	110
BEAN SALAD, canned		
(Green Giant)	½ cup	70
BEANS 'N FIXIN'S, canned (Hunt's)		
Big John's:		
Beans	3 oz.	100
Fixin's	1 oz.	50
BEAN SOUP (See SOUP, Bean)		
BEAN SPROUT:		
Mung, raw	½ lb.	80
Mung, boiled, drained	¼ lb.	32
Soy, raw	½ lb.	104
Soy, boiled, drained	¼ lb.	43
Canned (drained)	⅔ cup	6
BEAN, WHITE, canned		
(Goya) solids & liq.	½ cup	105
BEAN, YELLOW OR WAX:		
Boiled, 1″ pieces, drained	½ cup	18
Canned, regular pack, solids & liq.:		
(Del Monte) cut or french	½ cup	18

Food and Description	Measure or Quantity	Calories
(Larsen) *Freshlike*	½ cup	25
(Libby's) cut	4 oz.	23
(Stokely-Van Camp)	½ cup	23
Canned, dietetic (Featherweight) cut, solids & liq.	½ cup	25
Frozen (Frosty Acres)	3 oz.	25
BEAR CLAWS (Dolly Madison) cherry	2¾-oz. piece	270
BEEF, choice grade, medium done:		
Brisket, braised:		
Lean & fat	3 oz.	350
Lean only	3 oz.	189
Chuck, pot roast:		
Lean & fat	3 oz.	278
Lean only	3 oz.	182
Fat, separable, cooked	1 oz.	207
Filet mignon (See Steak, sirloin, lean)		
Flank, braised, 100% lean	3 oz.	167
Ground:		
Regular, raw	½ cup	303
Regular, broiled	3 oz.	243
Lean, broiled	3 oz.	186
Rib:		
Roasted, lean & fat	3 oz.	374
Lean only	3 oz.	205
Round:		
Broiled, lean & fat	3 oz.	222
Lean only	3 oz.	161
Rump:		
Broiled, lean & fat	3 oz.	295
Lean only	3 oz.	177
Steak, club, broiled:		
One 8-oz. steak (weighed without bone before cooking) will give you:		
Lean & fat	5.9 oz.	754
Lean only	3.4 oz.	234
Steak, porterhouse, broiled:		
One 16-oz. steak (weighed with bone before cooking) will give you:		
Lean & fat	10.2 oz.	1339
Lean only	5.9 oz.	372
Steak, ribeye, broiled:		
One 10-oz. steak (weighed without bone before cooking) will give you:		

Food and Description	Measure or Quantity	Calories
Lean & fat	7.3 oz.	911
Lean only	3.8 oz.	258
Steak, sirloin, double-bone, broiled:		
One 16-oz. steak (weighed with bone before cooking) will give you:		
Lean & fat	8.9 oz.	1028
Lean only	5.9 oz.	359
One 12-oz. steak (weighed with bone before cooking) will give you:		
Lean & fat	6.6 oz.	767
Lean only	4.4 oz.	268
Steak, T-bone, broiled:		
One 16-oz. steak (weighed with bone before cooking) will give you:		
Lean & fat	9.8 oz.	1315
Lean only	5.5 oz.	348
BEEFAMATO COCKTAIL, canned (Mott's)	6 fl. oz.	80
BEEF BOUILLON:		
Regular:		
(Herb-Ox):		
Cube	1 cube	6
Packet	1 packet	8
(Knorr)	1 cube	15
(Wyler's)	1 cube	6
Low sodium:		
(Borden) *Lite-Line*, instant	1 tsp.	12
(Featherweight)	1 tsp.	18
BEEF, CHIPPED:		
Cooked, home recipe	½ cup	188
Frozen, creamed:		
(Banquet) creamed	4-oz. pkg.	100
(Stouffer's)	5½-oz. serving	230
BEEF DINNER OR ENTREE:		
*Canned (Hunt's) oriental, *Entree Maker*	7.6 oz.	271
Frozen:		
(Armour):		
Classics Lite, Steak Diane	10-oz. meal	290
Dinner Classics, sirloin tips	10¼-oz. dinner	230
(Banquet):		
Dinner chopped	11-oz. dinner	420
Extra Helping	16-oz. dinner	870
Platter	10-oz. meal	460
(Healthy Choice) sirloin tips	11¾-oz. meal	290
(La Choy) Fresh & Light, & broccoli with rice	11-oz. meal	260
(Le Menu):		
Chopped sirloin	11½-oz. dinner	390

Food and Description	Measure or Quantity	Calories
Yankee pot roast	11-oz. dinner	360
(Morton) sliced	10-oz. dinner	220
(Stouffer's):		
Lean Cuisine, oriental with		
vegetables & rice	8⅝-oz. meal	250
Right Course:		
Dijon	9½-oz. meal	290
Fiesta	8⅞-oz. meal	270
(Swanson):		
Regular, 4-compartment, chopped		
sirloin	11½-oz. dinner	350
Hungry Man:		
Chopped	17¼-oz. dinner	600
Sliced	12¼-oz. entree	330
(Weight Watchers):		
London broil in mushroom sauce	7.37-oz. meal	140
Sirloin tips & mushrooms in		
wine sauce	7½-oz. meal	250
BEEF, DRIED, canned:		
(Hormel)	1 oz.	45
(Swift)	1 oz.	47
BEEF GOULASH (Hormel)		
Short Orders	7½-oz. can	230
BEEF, GROUND, SEASONING MIX:		
(Durkee):		
Regular	1 cup	653
With onion	1 cup	659
(French's) with onion	1⅛-oz. pkg.	100
BEEF HASH, ROAST:		
Canned, *Mary Kitchen* (Hormel):		
Regular	7½-oz. serving	350
Short Orders	7½-oz. can	360
Frozen (Stouffer's)	10-oz. meal	380
BEEF, PACKAGED		
(Carl Buddig)	1 oz.	40
BEEF, PEPPER ORIENTAL, frozen:		
(Chun King)	13-oz. meal	310
(La Choy) dinner	12-oz. dinner	250
BEEF PIE, frozen:		
(Banquet)	7-oz. pie	510
(Empire Kosher)	8-oz. pie	540
(Morton)	7-oz. pie	430
(Swanson):		
Regular	8-oz. pie	400
Chunky	10-oz. pie	530
BEEF PUFFS, frozen (Durkee)	1 piece	47
BEEF ROLL (Hormel) Lumberjack	1 oz.	101

Food and Description	Measure or Quantity	Calories
BEEF, SHORT RIBS, frozen:		
(Armour) *Dinner Classics,* boneless	9¾-oz. dinner	380
(Stouffer's) boneless, with gravy	9-oz. pkg.	350
BEEF SOUP (See SOUP, Beef)		
BEEF SPREAD, ROAST, canned (Underwood)	½ of 4¾-oz. can	140
BEEF STEAK, BREADED (Hormel) frozen	4-oz. serving	370
BEEF STEW:		
Home recipe, made with lean beef chuck	1 cup	218
Canned, regular pack:		
Dinty Moore (Hormel):		
Regular	8-oz. serving	210
Short Orders	7½-oz. can	150
(Libby's)	7½-oz. serving	160
Canned, dietetic (Estee)	7½-oz. serving	210
Frozen:		
(Banquet)	¼ of 28-oz. pkg.	140
(Stouffer's)	10-oz. serving	305
BEEF STEW SEASONING MIX:		
*(Durkee)	1 cup	379
(French's)	1 pkg.	150
BEEF STOCK BASE (French's)	1 tsp.	8
BEEF STROGANOFF, frozen:		
(Le Menu)	9¼ oz. dinner	430
(Stouffer's) with parsley noodles	9¾ oz.	390
(Weight Watchers)	9-oz. meal	320
*BEEF STROGANOFF SEASONING MIX (Durkee)	1 cup	820
BEER & ALE:		
Regular:		
Anheuser	8 fl. oz.	139
Black Horse Ale	8 fl. oz.	108
Black Label (Heilemann)	8 fl. oz.	68
Blatz (Heilemann)	8 fl. oz.	93
Budweiser	8 fl. oz.	118
Carlsberg	8 fl. oz.	100
Michelob, regular	8 fl. oz.	113
Old Milwaukee	8 fl. oz.	95
Pearl Premium	8 fl. oz.	99
Schlitz	8 fl. oz.	100
Stroh Bohemian	8 fl. oz.	84
Light or low carbohydrate:		
Bud Dry	8 fl. oz.	87
Budweiser, light	8 fl. oz.	73
Busch, light	8 fl. oz.	73

Food and Description	Measure or Quantity	Calories
Carlsberg, light	8 fl. oz.	73
C. Schmidt's, light	8 fl. oz.	64
LA	8 fl. oz.	75
Michelob, dry	8 fl. oz.	88
Natural Light	8 fl. oz.	73
Special Export Light	8 fl. oz.	76
BEER, NEAR:		
Goetz Pale	8 fl. oz.	53
(Metbrew)	8 fl. oz.	49
BEET:		
Boiled, whole	2"-dia. beet	16
Boiled, sliced	½ cup	33
Canned, regular pack, solids & liq.:		
(Blue Boy) Harvard	½ cup	100
(Del Monte):		
Pickled	4 oz.	77
Sliced	4 oz.	29
(Greenwood):		
Harvard	½ cup	70
Pickled	½ cup	110
(Larsen) *Freshlike:*		
Regular	½ cup	40
Pickled	½ cup	100
(Stokely-Van Camp) pickled	½ cup	95
Canned, dietetic, solids & liq.:		
(Blue Boy) whole	½ cup	39
(Comstock)	½ cup	30
(Featherweight) sliced	½ cup	45
(Larsen) *Fresh-Lite*	½ cup	40
(S&W) *Nutradiet,* sliced	½ cup	35
BEET PUREE, canned (Larsen)	½ cup	45
BENEDICTINE LIQUEUR (Julius Wile)	1½ fl. oz.	168
BERRY BEARS, *Fruit Corners,* assorted or fruit punch	.9-oz. pkg.	100
BERRY CITRUS DRINK (Five Alive), chilled or *frozen	6 fl. oz.	88
BERRY DRINK:		
Canned, *Ssips* (Johanna Farms)	8.45-fl. oz. container	130
*Mix, dietetic, *Crystal Light*	8 fl. oz.	3
BIGG MIXX, cereal (Kellogg's):		
Plain	½ cup (1 oz.)	110
With raisins	½ cup (1.3 oz.)	140
BIG MAC (See *McDONALD'S*)		
BISCUIT DOUGH (Pillsbury):		
Baking Powder, *1869 Brand*	1 biscuit	100
Buttermilk:		
Regular	1 biscuit	50

Food and Description	Measure or Quantity	Calories
Ballard, *Oven Ready*	1 biscuit	50
Extra rich, *Hungry Jack*	1 biscuit	50
Fluffy, *Hungry Jack*	1 biscuit	90
Butter Tastin', *1869 Brand*	1 biscuit	100
Flaky, *Hungry Jack*, regular	1 biscuit	80
Oven Ready, Ballard	1 biscuit	50
BITTERS (Angostura)	1 tsp.	14
BLACKBERRY, fresh, hulled	1 cup	84
BLACKBERRY JELLY:		
Sweetened (Home Brands)	1 T.	14
Dietetic:		
(Diet Delight)	1 T.	12
(Featherweight)	1 T.	16
BLACKBERRY LIQUEUR (Bols)	1 fl. oz.	95
BLACKBERRY PRESERVE OR JAM:		
Sweetened (Smucker's)	1 T.	53
Dietetic:		
(Estee; Louis Sherry)	1 T.	6
(Featherweight)	1 T.	16
(S&W) *Nutradiet*	1 T.	12
BLACKBERRY WINE (Mogen David)	3 fl. oz.	135
BLACK-EYED PEAS:		
Canned:		
(Allen's)	½ cup	100
(Goya)	½ cup	105
(Green Giant)	½ cup	90
(Trappey's) any style	½ cup	90
Frozen:		
(Birds Eye)	⅓ pkg.	133
(Frosty Acres)	3.3 oz.	130
(McKenzie; Seabrook Farms)	⅓ pkg.	130
(Southland)	⅕ of 16-oz. pkg.	130
BLINTZ, frozen:		
(Empire Kosher):		
Apple	2½ oz.	100
Blueberry & cheese	2½ oz.	110
Potato	2½ oz.	130
(King Kold) cheese	2½ oz.	132
BLOODY MARY MIX:		
Dry (Bar-Tender's)	1 serving	26
Liquid:		
(Holland House) *Smooth 'N Spicy*	6 fl. oz.	18
(Libby's)	6 fl. oz.	40
Tabasco	6 fl. oz.	56
Liquid (Sacramento)	5½-fl.-oz. can	39
BLUEBERRY, fresh, whole	½ cup	45

Food and Description	Measure or Quantity	Calories
BLUEBERRY PIE (See PIE, Blueberry)		
BLUEBERRY PRESERVE OR JAM:		
Sweetened:		
(Home Brands)	1 T.	52
(Smucker's)	1 T.	54
Dietetic (Louis Sherry)	1 T.	6
BLUEFISH, broiled	3½" × 3" × ½" piece	199
BODY BUDDIES, cereal (General Mills), natural fruit flavor	¾ cup	110
BOLOGNA:		
(Eckrich):		
Beef:		
Regular, garlic	1 oz.	90
Thick slice	1½-oz. slice	140
German brand	1-oz. slice	80
Meat, regular	1-oz. slice	90
(Hebrew National) beef	1 oz.	90
(Hormel):		
Beef	1-oz. slice	85
Meat	1-oz. slice	90
(Ohse):		
Regular	1 oz.	85
15% chicken	1 oz.	90
(Oscar Mayer):		
Beef	.5-oz. slice	48
Beef	1-oz. slice	90
Beef Lebanon	.8-oz. slice	47
Garlic beef	1-oz. slice	90
Meat	1-oz. slice	90
(Swift) *Light & Lean*	1-oz. slice	95
BOLOGNA & CHEESE:		
(Eckrich)	.7-oz. slice	90
(Oscar Mayer)	.8-oz. slice	74
BONITO, canned (Star-Kist):		
Chunk	6½-oz. can	605
Solid	7-oz. can	650
BOO*BERRY, cereal (General Mills)	1 cup	110
BORSCHT, canned:		
Regular:		
(Gold's)	8-oz. serving	100
(Manischewitz) with beets	8-oz. serving	80
(Mother's) old fashioned	8-oz. serving	90
Dietetic or low calorie:		
(Gold's)	8-oz. serving	20
(Manischewitz)	8-oz. serving	20
(Mother's):		
Artificially sweetened	8-oz. serving	29

Food and Description	Measure or Quantity	Calories
Unsalted	8-oz. serving	107
(Rokeach):		
Diet	8-oz. serving	15
Unsalted	8-oz. serving	103
BOSCO (See SYRUP)		
BOUILLON (See specific flavor)		
BOURBON (See DISTILLED LIQUOR)		
BOYSENBERRY JELLY:		
Sweetened (Home Brands)	1 T.	15
Dietetic (S&W) *Nutradiet,* red label	1 T.	12
BOYSENBERRY JUICE, canned (Smucker's)	8 fl. oz.	120
BRAN:		
Crude	1 oz.	60
Miller's (Elam's)	1 oz.	87
BRAN BREAKFAST CEREAL:		
(Kellogg's):		
All Bran or *Bran Buds*	⅓ cup	70
Cracklin' Oat Bran	½ cup	110
Fruitful Bran	⅔ cup	110
Oat bran, *Common Sense,* with raisins	½ cup	120
(Loma Linda)	1 oz.	90
(Malt-O-Meal) raisin	¾ cup	129
(Nabisco)	½ cup	70
(Post) flakes	⅔ cup	88
(Ralston Purina):		
Bran Chex	⅔ cup	90
Oat	1 cup	130
BRANDY (See DISTILLED LIQUOR)		
BRANDY, FLAVORED		
(Mr. Boston):		
Apricot	1 fl. oz.	94
Blackberry	1 fl. oz.	92
Cherry	1 fl. oz.	87
Ginger	1 fl. oz.	72
Peach	1 fl. oz.	94
BRAUNSCHWEIGER:		
(Eckrich) chub	1 oz.	70
(Oscar Mayer) chub	1 oz.	94
(Swift) 8-oz. chub	1 oz.	109
BRAZIL NUT:		
Shelled	4 nuts	114
Roasted (Fisher) salted	1 oz.	193
BREAD, REGULAR:		
Apple cinnamon (Pritikin)	1-oz. slice	80
Autumn grain, *Merita*	1-oz. slice	75

Food and Description	Measure or Quantity	Calories
Barbecue, *Millbrook*	1.23-oz. slice	100
Boston Brown	3″ × ¾″ slice	101
Bran (Roman Meal):		
5 Bran	1-oz. slice	65
Oat, light	.8-oz. slice	42
Rice, honey	1-oz. slice	71
Bran'nola (Arnold)	1.3-oz. slice	90
Buttermilk:		
Butternut or Holsum	1-oz. slice	80
Sweetheart	1-oz. slice	70
Cinnamon (Pepperidge Farm)	.9-oz. slice	85
Cracked wheat:		
(Pepperidge Farm)	.9-oz. slice	70
(Roman Meal)	1-oz. slice	67
Crispbread, *Wasa:*		
Rye, lite	.3-oz. slice	30
Sesame	.5-oz. slice	50
Date-nut roll (Dromedary)	1-oz. slice	80
Egg, *Millbrook*	1-oz. slice	70
Flatbread, *Ideal:*		
Bran	.2-oz. slice	19
Extra thin	1-oz. slice	12
Whole grain	.2-oz. slice	19
French:		
Eddy's, regular or sour	1-oz. slice	70
Francisco (Arnold)	1-oz. slice	70
(Wonder)	1-oz. slice	71
Garlic (Arnold)	1-oz. slice	80
Hi-Fibre (Monk's)	1-oz. slice	50
Hillbilly, Holsum	1-oz. slice	70
Hollywood, dark	1-oz. slice	70
Honey bran (Pepperidge Farm)	1-oz. slice	95
Honey wheat berry (Arnold)	1.1-oz. slice	80
Hunters Grain, *Country Farms*	1.5-oz. slice	120
Italian (Arnold) *Francisco*	1 slice	70
Low sodium, *Butternut*	1-oz. slice	80
Multi-grain:		
(Arnold) *Milk & Honey*	1-oz. slice	70
Country Farms	1-oz. slice	80
(Pritikin)	1-oz. slice	70
(Weight Watchers)	.74-oz. slice	40
Natural grains (Arnold)	.8-oz. slice	60
Oat:		
(Arnold) *Milk & Honey*	1-oz. slice	80
(Weight Watchers)	.74-oz. slice	39
Oatmeal (Pepperidge Farm)	.9-oz. slice	70
Olympic Meal, *Holsum*	1-oz. slice	70
Onion dill (Pritikin)	1-oz. slice	70

Food and Description	Measure or Quantity	Calories
Pita (see *Sahara*, Thomas')		
Protein (Thomas')	.7-oz. slice	46
Pumpernickel:		
(Arnold)	1-oz. slice	80
(Levy's)	1.1-oz. slice	80
(Pepperidge Farm):		
Regular	1.1-oz. slice	80
Party	.2-oz. slice	17
Raisin:		
(Arnold) tea	.9-oz. slice	70
(Monk's) & cinnamon	1-oz. slice	70
(Pepperidge Farm)	1 slice	75
(Pritikin)	1-oz. slice	70
(Sun-Maid)	1-oz. slice	80
(Weight Watchers)	.8-oz. slice	49
Rye:		
(Arnold) Jewish	1.1-oz. slice	80
(Levy's) real	1.1-oz. slice	80
(Pepperidge Farm) family	1.1-oz. slice	85
(Pritikin)	1-oz. slice	70
(Weight Watchers)	.74-oz. slice	39
(Wonder)	1-oz. slice	70
Sahara (Thomas') wheat or white	1-oz. piece	80
Sandwich (Roman Meal)	.8-oz. slice	56
7 Grain (Roman Meal) light	.8-oz. slice	40
Sourdough, *Di Carlo*	1-oz. slice	70
Sunflower & bran (Monk's)	1-oz. slice	70
Wheat (see also Cracked Wheat or Whole Wheat):		
America's Own, cottage	1-oz. slice	70
(Arnold):		
Bran'nola	1.3-oz. slice	80
Less or *Liteway*	.8-oz. slice	40
Milk & Honey	1-oz. slice	80
Fresh Horizons	1-oz. slice	50
Fresh & Natural	1-oz. slice	70
Home Pride	1-oz. slice	70
(Pepperidge Farm) sandwich	.8-oz. slice	55
(Roman Meal)	.8-oz. slice	40
(Weight Watchers)	.74-oz. slice	40
Wheatberry, *Home Pride*, honey	1-oz. slice	70
White:		
America's Own, cottage	1-oz. slice	70
(Arnold):		
Brick Oven	.8-oz. slice	60
Country	1.3-oz. slice	100
Less	.8-oz. slice	40
Milk & Honey	1-oz. slice	80
Home Pride	1-oz. slice	72

Food and Description	Measure or Quantity	Calories
(Monk's)	1-oz. slice	60
(Pepperidge Farm):		
Regular	1.2-oz. slice	75
Toasting	1.2-oz. slice	85
(Wonder) regular	1-oz. slice	70
Wholegrain (Roman Meal)	1-oz. slice	63
Whole wheat:		
(Arnold) *Stone Ground*	.8-oz. slice	50
(Monk's)	1-oz. slice	70
(Pepperidge Farm) thin slice	1 slice	65
(Roman Meal)	1-oz. slice	67
BREAD, CANNED, brown, plain or raisin (B&M)	½" slice	80
BREAD CRUMBS:		
(Contadina) seasoned	½ cup	211
(4C) any type	1 T.	35
(Pepperidge Farm)	1 oz.	110
***BREAD DOUGH:**		
Frozen:		
(Pepperidge Farm):		
Country rye or white	⅒ loaf	80
Stone ground wheat	⅒ loaf	75
(Rich's):		
French	1/20 loaf	59
Italian	1/20 loaf	60
Refrigerated (Pillsbury):		
French	1" slice	60
Wheat or white	1" slice	80
***BREAD MIX:**		
Home Hearth:		
French	⅜" slice	85
Rye or white	⅜" slice	75
(Pillsbury):		
Banana	1/12 loaf	170
Cherry nut	1/12 loaf	180
BREAD PUDDING, with raisins, home recipe	½ cup	248
BREAD STICK (Stella D'Oro):		
Plain or onion	1 piece	40
Sesame	1 piece	50
***BREAD STICK DOUGH** (Pillsbury)	1 piece	100
***BREAKFAST DRINK** (Pillsbury)	1 pouch	290
BREAKFAST SQUARES (General Mills) all flavors	1 bar	190
BRITOS, frozen (Patio):		
Beef & bean, chicken, spicy or green chili	3.6-oz. serving	250
Nacho beef	3.6-oz. serving	270

Food and Description	Measure or Quantity	Calories
BROCCOLI:		
Boiled, with stalk	1 stalk (6.3 oz.)	47
Boiled, ½" pieces	½ cup	20
Frozen:		
(Birds Eye):		
In cheese sauce	5 oz.	132
Chopped, cuts or florets	⅓ pkg.	26
(Frosty Acres)	3.3 oz.	25
(Green Giant):		
Cuts:		
In cream sauce:		
Regular	⅓ of 10-oz. pkg.	50
One Serving	5-oz. pkg.	70
Harvest Fresh	3 oz.	16
Polybag	½ cup	12
Spears:		
In butter sauce, regular	⅓ of 10-oz. serving	40
Harvest Fresh	3 oz.	19
(Larsen)	3.3 oz.	25
(Seabrook Farms) chopped or spears	⅓ of 10-oz. pkg.	30
(Stouffer's) in cheese sauce	½ of 9-oz. pkg.	130
BROTH & SEASONING:		
(George Washington)	1 packet	5
Maggi	1 T.	22
BRUNSWICK STEW, canned (Hormel) *Short Orders*	7½-oz. can	220
BRUSSELS SPROUT:		
Boiled	3–4 sprouts	28
Frozen:		
(Birds Eye):		
Regular	⅓ pkg.	37
Baby, with cheese sauce	4½ oz.	128
(Frosty Acres)	3.3 oz.	35
(Green Giant):		
In butter sauce	3.3 oz.	40
Polybag	½ cup	25
BUCKWHEAT, cracked (Pocono)	1 oz.	104
BUC*WHEATS, cereal (General Mills)	1 oz. (¾ cup)	110
BULGUR, canned, seasoned	4 oz.	206
BURGER KING:		
Apple pie	1 serving	305
Breakfast bagel sandwich:		
Plain	1 sandwich	387
Ham	1 sandwich	418
Sausage	1 sandwich	621
Breakfast Croissan'wich:		
Bacon	1 serving	355

Food and Description	Measure or Quantity	Calories
Ham	1 serving	335
Sausage	1 serving	538
Cheeseburger:		
Regular	1 serving	304
Double:		
Plain	1 serving	464
With bacon	1 serving	510
Condiments:		
Ketchup	1 serving on burger	11
Mustard	1 serving on burger	2
Pickles	1 serving on burger	0
Chicken specialty sandwich:		
Plain	1 serving	492
Condiments:		
Lettuce	1 serving on sandwich	2
Mayonnaise	1 serving on sandwich	94
Chicken Tenders	1 piece	34
Coffee, regular	1 serving	2
Danish	1 piece	500
Egg platter, scrambled:		
Bacon	1 serving	68
Croissant	1 serving	187
Eggs	1 serving	119
Hash browns	1 serving	162
Sausage	1 serving	234
French fries	1 regular order	227
French toast sticks	1 serving	499
Hamburger:		
Plain	1 burger	262
Condiments:		
Ketchup	1 serving on burger	11
Mustard	1 serving on burger	2
Pickles	1 serving on burger	0
Ham & cheese specialty:		
Plain	1 sandwich	365
Condiments:		
Lettuce	1 serving on sandwich	2
Mayonnaise	1 serving on sandwich	94
Tomato	1 serving on sandwich	6
Milk:		
2% low fat	1 serving	121

Food and Description	Measure or Quantity	Calories
Whole	1 serving	157
Onion rings	1 serving	274
Orange juice	1 serving	82
Salad:		
Chef	1 salad	180
Chicken	1 salad	140
Side	1 salad	20
Salad dressing:		
Regular:		
Bleu cheese	1 serving	156
House	1 serving	130
1000 Island	1 serving	117
Dietetic, Italian	1 serving	14
Shakes:		
Chocolate	1 shake	374
Vanilla	1 shake	334
Soft drink:		
Sweetened:		
Pepsi-Cola	1 regular size	159
7-UP	1 regular size	144
Diet *Pepsi*	1 regular size	1
Whaler:		
Plain sandwich	1 sandwich	353
Condiments:		
Lettuce	1 serving on sandwich	1
Tartar sauce	1 serving on sandwich	134
Whopper:		
Regular:		
Plain	1 sandwich	452
With cheese	1 sandwich	535
Condiments:		
Ketchup	1 serving on sandwich	17
Lettuce	1 serving on sandwich	1
Mayonnaise	1 serving on sandwich	146
Onion	1 serving on sandwich	5
Pickles	1 serving on sandwich	1
Tomato	1 serving on sandwich	6
Junior:		
Plain	1 sandwich	262
With cheese	1 sandwich	305

Food and Description	Measure or Quantity	Calories
Condiments:		
Ketchup	1 serving on sandwich	8
Lettuce	1 serving on sandwich	1
Mayonnaise	1 serving on sandwich	48
Pickles	1 serving on sandwich	0
Tomato	1 serving on sandwich	3
BURGUNDY WINE:		
(Louis M. Martini)	3 fl. oz.	60
(Paul Masson)	3 fl. oz.	70
(Taylor)	3 fl. oz.	75
BURGUNDY WINE, SPARKLING:		
(Carlo Rossi)	3 fl. oz.	69
(Great Western)	3 fl. oz.	82
(Taylor)	3 fl. oz.	78
BURRITO:		
*Canned (Old El Paso)	1 burrito	299
Frozen:		
(Hormel):		
Beef	1 burrito	220
Cheese	1 burrito	250
Hot chili	1 burrito	210
(Fred's) *Little Juan:*		
Bean & cheese	5-oz. serving	331
Beef & potato	5-oz. serving	389
Chili, red	10-oz. serving	799
Red hot	5-oz. serving	433
(Old El Paso):		
Regular:		
Bean & cheese	1 piece	340
Beef & bean, mild	1 piece	330
Dinner, beef & bean	11-oz. dinner	470
(Patio):		
Beef & bean, regular	5-oz. meal	370
Red hot	5-oz. meal	360
(Swanson) bran & beef	15¼-oz. meal	720
(Van de Kamp's) regular crispy fried	6-oz. serving	365
(Weight Watchers) beefsteak or chicken	7.6-oz. meal	310
BURRITO FILLING MIX, canned		
(Del Monte)	½ cup	110
BURRITO SEASONING MIX		
(Lawry's)	1 pkg.	132

Food and Description	Measure or Quantity	Calories
BUTTER:		
Regular:		
(Breakstone)	1 T.	100
(Meadow Gold)	1 tsp.	35
Whipped (Land O'Lakes)	1 T.	75
BUTTER SUBSTITUTE, *Butter Buds:*		
Dry or liquid	⅛ oz. dry or 1 oz. liq.	12
Sprinkles	1 tsp.	14
BUTTERSCOTCH MORSELS		
(Nestlé)	1 oz.	150

C

Food and Description	Measure or Quantity	Calories
CABBAGE:		
Boiled, until tender, without salt, drained	1 cup	29
Canned, solids & liq.:		
(Comstock) red	½ cup	60
(Greenwood)	½ cup	60
Frozen (Stouffer's) stuffed with meat, *Lean Cuisine*	10¾-oz. meal	220
CABERNET SAUVIGNON:		
(Louis M. Martini):		
Napa Valley or Sonoma County	3 fl. oz.	61
Vineyard Selection	3 fl. oz.	67
(Paul Masson)	3 fl. oz.	70
CAFE COMFORT, 55 proof	1 fl. oz.	79
CAKE:		
Regular, non-frozen:		
Plain, home recipe, with butter, with boiled white icing	⅑ of 9″ square	401
Angel food:		
Home recipe	¹⁄₁₂ of 8″ cake	108
(Dolly Madison)	⅙ of 10½-oz. cake	120
Apple (Dolly Madison) dutch, *Buttercrunch*	1½-oz. piece	170
Apple spice (Entenmann's) fat & cholesterol free	1-oz. slice	80
Banana crunch (Entenmann's) fat & cholesterol free	1-oz. slice	80
Blueberry crunch (Entenmann's) fat & cholesterol free	1-oz. slice	70
Butter streusel (Dolly Madison) *Buttercrumb*	1½-oz. piece	150
Caramel, home recipe, with caramel icing	⅑ of 9″ square	322
Carrot (Dolly Madison) *Lunch Cake*	3¼-oz. serving	350
Chocolate, home recipe, with chocolate icing, 2-layer	¹⁄₁₂ of 9″ cake	365
Chocolate (Dolly Madison)		

28

Food and Description	Measure or Quantity	Calories
German, *Lunch Cake*	3½-oz. piece	440
Chocolate loaf (Entenmann's) fat & cholesterol free	1-oz. slice	70
Cinnamon (Dolly Madison) *Buttercrumb*	1½-oz. piece	170
Creme (Dolly Madison) *Lunch Cake*	⅞-oz. cake	90
Cinnamon (Dolly Madison) butter		
Coffee (Entenmann's) fat & cholesterol free, chewy or cinnamon apple	1.3-oz. piece	90
Fruit:		
Home recipe, dark	⅓₀ of 8" loaf	57
Home recipe, made with butter	⅓₀ of 8" loaf	58
(Holland Honey Cake) unsalted	¹⁄₁₄ of cake	80
Golden (Entenmann's) loaf, fat & cholesterol free	1-oz. slice	80
Hawaiian spice (Dolly Madison) *Lunch Cake*	3½-oz. pkg.	350
Honey 'n spice (Dolly Madison)	3¼-oz. serving	330
Pineapple crunch (Entenmann's) fat & cholesterol free	1-oz. slice	70
Pound, home recipe, traditional, made with butter	3½" × 3½" slice	123
Raisin date loaf (Holland Honey Cake) low sodium	¹⁄₁₄ of 13-oz. cake	8
Sponge, home recipe	¹⁄₁₂ of 10" cake	196
White, home recipe, made with butter, without icing, 2-layer	⅑ of 9" wide, 3" high cake	353
White (Dolly Madison) coconut layer	¹⁄₁₂ of 30-oz. cake	220
Yellow, home recipe, made with butter, without icing, 2-layer	¹⁄₁₉ of cake	351
Frozen:		
Black forest (Weight Watchers)	3-oz. serving	180
Boston cream (Weight Watchers)	3-oz. serving	190
Butterscotch pecan (Pepperidge Farm) layer	¹⁄₁₀ of 17-oz. cake	160
Carrot:		
(Pepperidge Farm)	⅛ of 11¾-oz. cake	140
(Weight Watchers)	3-oz. serving	170
Cheesecake:		
(Morton) *Great Little Desserts:*		
Cherry	6-oz. cake	460
Cream cheese	6-oz. cake	480
Strawberry	6-oz. cake	470
(Rich's) Viennese	¹⁄₁₄ of 42-oz. cake	230

29

Food and Description	Measure or Quantity	Calories
(Weight Watchers):		
Regular	3.9-oz. serving	220
Strawberry	3.9-oz. serving	180
Chocolate:		
(Pepperidge Farm):		
Layer, fudge	1/10 of 17-oz. cake	180
Supreme, regular	1/4 of 11½-oz. cake	310
(Weight Watchers) German	2½ oz.	190
Coconut (Pepperidge Farm) layer	1/10 of 17-oz. cake	180
Crumb (See ROLL OR BUN, Crumb)		
Devil's food (Pepperidge Farm) layer	1/10 of 17-oz. cake	180
Golden (Pepperidge Farm) layer	1/10 of 17-oz. cake	180
Grand Marnier (Pepperidge Farm)	1½ oz.	160
Lemon coconut (Pepperidge Farm)	1/4 of 12¼-oz. cake	280
Pound, (Pepperidge Farm) butter	1/10 of 10¾-oz.cake	130
Strawberry cream (Pepperidge Farm) Supreme	1/12 of 12-oz. cake	190
Vanilla (Pepperidge Farm) layer	1/10 of 17-oz. cake	180
CAKE OR COOKIE ICING		
(Pillsbury):		
All flavors except chocolate	1 T.	70
Chocolate	1 T.	60
CAKE ICING:		
Amaretto almond (Betty Crocker) *Creamy Deluxe*	1/12 can	160
Butter pecan (Betty Crocker) *Creamy Deluxe*	1/12 can	170
Caramel, home recipe	4 oz.	408
Caramel pecan (Pillsbury) *Frosting Supreme*	1/12 can	160
Cherry (Betty Crocker) *Creamy Deluxe*	1/12 can	160
Chocolate:		
(Betty Crocker) *Creamy Deluxe:*		
Regular, with candy-coated chocolate chips, with dinosaurs, milk or sour cream	1/12 can	160
Chips	1/12 can	152
(Duncan Hines):		
Fudge, dark dutch	1/12 can	149
Milk	1/12 can	151
(Pillsbury) *Frosting Supreme,* fudge, nut or milk	1/12 can	150

Food and Description	Measure or Quantity	Calories
Coconut almond (Pillsbury) *Frosting Supreme*	⅟₁₂ can	150
Cream cheese:		
(Betty Crocker) *Creamy Deluxe*	⅟₁₂ can	160
(Duncan Hines)	⅟₁₂ can	152
(Pillsbury) *Frosting Supreme*	⅟₁₂ can	160
Double dutch (Pillsbury) *Frosting Supreme*	⅟₁₂ can	140
Lemon (Pillsbury) *Frosting Supreme*	⅟₁₂ can	160
Polka dot (Duncan Hines) pink vanilla	⅟₁₂ can	154
Rainbow chip (Betty Crocker) *Creamy Deluxe*	⅟₁₂ can	170
Rocky road (Betty Crocker) *Creamy Deluxe*	⅟₁₂ can	150
Strawberry (Pillsbury) *Frosting Supreme*	⅟₁₂ can	160
Vanilla:		
(Betty Crocker) *Creamy Deluxe*	⅟₁₂ can	160
(Duncan Hines)	⅟₁₂ can	151
(Pillsbury) *Frosting Supreme*, regular or sour cream	⅟₁₂ can	160
White:		
Home recipe, boiled	4 oz.	358
Home recipe, uncooked	4 oz.	426
(Betty Crocker) *Creamy Deluxe*	⅟₁₂ can	160
*CAKE ICING MIX:		
Regular:		
Chocolate:		
Home recipe, fudge	½ cup	586
(Betty Crocker) creamy:		
Fudge	⅟₁₂ pkg.	180
Milk	⅟₁₂ pkg.	170
(Pillsbury) *Frost It Hot*	⅛ pkg.	50
Coconut almond (Pillsbury)	⅟₁₂ pkg.	160
Coconut pecan:		
(Betty Crocker) creamy	⅟₁₂ pkg.	150
(Pillsbury)	⅟₁₂ pkg.	150
Lemon (Betty Crocker) creamy	⅟₁₂ pkg.	180
Vanilla (Betty Crocker) creamy	⅟₁₂ pkg.	170
White:		
(Betty Crocker) fluffy	⅟₁₂ pkg.	70
(Betty Crocker) sour cream, creamy	⅟₁₂ pkg.	170
(Pillsbury) fluffy:		
Regular	⅟₁₂ pkg.	60
Frost It Hot	⅛ pkg.	50

Food and Description	Measure or Quantity	Calories
Dietetic:		
(Estee)	1½ tsp.	50
(Pritikin) *Frostlite*	¹⁄₁₂ pkg.	25
CAKE MEAL (Manischewitz)	½ cup	286
CAKE MIX:		
Regular:		
Angel Food:		
(Betty Crocker):		
Confetti, lemon custard or white	¹⁄₁₂ pkg.	150
Traditional	¹⁄₁₂ pkg.	130
(Duncan Hines)	¹⁄₁₂ pkg.	131
*Apple streusel (Betty Crocker) *MicroRave*:		
Regular	⅙ of cake	240
No cholesterol recipe	⅙ of cake	210
*Banana (Pillsbury) *Pillsbury Plus*	¹⁄₁₂ of cake	250
*Boston cream (Pillsbury) *Bundt*	¹⁄₁₆ of cake	270
*Butter (Pillsbury) *Pillsbury Plus*	¹⁄₁₂ of cake	260
*Butter Brickle (Betty Crocker) *Supermoist*:		
Regular	¹⁄₁₂ of cake	250
No cholesterol recipe	¹⁄₁₂ of cake	220
*Butter pecan (Betty Crocker) *Supermoist*	¹⁄₁₂ of cake	250
*Carrot (Betty Crocker) *Supermoist*:		
Regular	¹⁄₁₂ of cake	250
No cholesterol recipe	¹⁄₁₂ of cake	220
*Carrot'n spice (Pillsbury) *Pillsbury Plus*	¹⁄₁₂ of cake	260
*Cheesecake:		
(Jell-O)	⅛ of 8″ cake	283
(Royal) No Bake:		
Lite	⅛ of cake	210
Real	⅛ of cake	280
*Cherry chip (Betty Crocker) *Supermoist*	¹⁄₁₂ of cake	190
Chocolate:		
(Betty Crocker):		
**MicroRave*:		
Fudge, with vanilla frosting	⅙ of cake	310
German, with coconut pecan frosting	⅙ of cake	320
*Pudding	⅙ of cake	230
**Supermoist*:		
Chip:		
Regular	¹⁄₁₂ of cake	280

Food and Description	Measure or Quantity	Calories
No cholesterol recipe	¹⁄₁₂ of cake	220
Chocolate chip	¹⁄₁₂ of cake	260
Fudge	¹⁄₁₂ of cake	260
Sour cream:		
Regular	¹⁄₁₂ of cake	260
No cholesterol recipe	¹⁄₁₂ of cake	220
(Duncan Hines) fudge	¹⁄₁₂ pkg.	187
*(Pillsbury):		
Bundt, tunnel of fudge	¹⁄₁₆ of cake	260
Microwave:		
Plain	⅛ of cake	210
With chocolate frosting	⅛ of cake	300
Pillsbury Plus:		
Chocolate Chip	¹⁄₁₂ of cake	270
Dark	¹⁄₁₂ of cake	250
German	¹⁄₁₂ of cake	250
*Cinnamon (Pillsbury)		
Streusel Swirl, microwave	⅛ of cake	240
*Cinnamon pecan streusel (Betty Crocker) *MicroRave:*		
Regular	⅙ of cake	290
No cholesterol recipe	⅙ of cake	240
Coffee cake:		
*(Aunt Jemima)	⅛ of cake	170
*(Pillsbury) Apple cinnamon	⅛ of cake	240
Devil's food:		
*(Betty Crocker):		
MicroRave, with chocolate frosting:		
Regular	⅙ of cake	310
No cholesterol recipe	⅙ of cake	240
Supermoist:		
Regular	¹⁄₁₂ of cake	260
No cholesterol recipe	¹⁄₁₂ of cake	220
(Duncan Hines) deluxe	¹⁄₁₂ pkg.	189
*(Pillsbury) *Pillsbury Plus*	¹⁄₁₂ of cake	270
Fudge (See Chocolate)		
Golden (Duncan Hines) butter recipe	¹⁄₁₂ pkg.	188
Lemon:		
(Betty Crocker) *Supermoist*	¹⁄₁₂ of cake	260
*(Pillsbury):		
Bundt, tunnel of	¹⁄₁₆ of cake	270
Streusel Swirl	¹⁄₁₆ of cake	270
*Lemon blueberry (Pillsbury) *Bundt*	¹⁄₁₆ of cake	200
*Marble (Betty Crocker) *Supermoist:*		
Regular	¹⁄₁₂ of cake	250
No cholesterol recipe	¹⁄₁₂ of cake	210

Food and Description	Measure or Quantity	Calories
*Pineapple creme (Pillsbury) *Bundt*	1/16 of cake	260
Pound:		
*(Betty Crocker) golden	1/12 of cake	200
*(Dromedary)	1/2" slice	150
*Rainbow chip (Betty Crocker) *Supermoist*	1/12 of cake	250
*Spice (Betty Crocker) *Supermoist:*		
Regular	1/12 of cake	260
No cholesterol recipe	1/12 of cake	220
Strawberry,		
*(Pillsbury) *Pillsbury Plus*	1/12 of cake	260
*Upside down (Betty Crocker) pineapple:		
Regular	1/9 of cake	250
No cholesterol recipe	1/9 of cake	240
*Vanilla (Betty Crocker) golden:		
MicroRave	1/6 of cake	320
Supermoist, regular	1/12 of cake	280
White:		
*(Betty Crocker) *Supermoist*:		
Regular	1/12 of cake	240
Sour cream	1/12 of cake	180
(Duncan Hines) deluxe	1/12 pkg.	188
Yellow:		
*(Betty Crocker):		
MicroRave, with chocolate frosting:		
Regular	1/6 of cake	300
No cholesterol recipe	1/6 of cake	230
Supermoist:		
Regular	1/12 of cake	260
No cholesterol recipe	1/12 of cake	220
(Duncan Hines) deluxe	1/12 pkg.	188
*(Pillsbury):		
*Microwave, plain	1/8 of cake	220
Pillsbury Plus	1/12 of cake	260
*Dietetic:		
(Estee) any flavor	1/10 of cake	100
(Pritikin) *Batterlite,* unfrosted	1/10 of cake	90
CAMPARI, 45 proof	1 fl. oz.	66
CANDY, REGULAR:		
Almond, Jordan (Banner)	1¼-oz. box	154
Almond Joy (Hershey's)	1.76-oz. bar	250
Apricot Delight (Sahadi)	1 oz.	100
Baby Ruth	2-oz. piece	260
Bar None (Hershey's)	1½ oz.	240

Food and Description	Measure or Quantity	Calories
Bit-O-Honey (Nestlé)	1 oz.	120
Bonkers! any flavor	1 piece	20
Breath Savers (Life Savers)	1 piece	8
Butterfinger	2-oz. bar	260
Butternut (Hollywood Brands)	2¼-oz. bar	310
Caramel:		
Caramel Flipper (Wayne)	1 oz.	128
Caramel Nip (Pearson)	1 piece	30
Caramello (Hershey's)	1.6-oz. bar	220
Charleston Chew	2-oz. piece	240
Cherry, chocolate-covered		
(*Welch's*) dark	1 piece	90
Chocolate bar:		
Alpine white (Nestlé)	1 oz.	170
Brazil nut (Cadbury's)	2 oz.	310
Caramello (Cadbury's)	2 oz.	280
Crunch (Nestlé)	1¹⁄₁₆-oz. bar	160
Hazelnut (Cadbury's)	2 oz.	310
Milk:		
(Cadbury's)	2 oz.	300
(Hershey's)	1.55-oz. bar	240
(Nestlé)	.35-oz. bar	53
(Nestlé)	1¹⁄₁₆-oz. bar	159
Special Dark (Hershey's)	1.45-oz. bar	220
Chocolate bar with almonds:		
(Cadbury's)	2 oz.	310
(Hershey's):		
Regular	1.45-oz. bar	230
Golden Almond	3.2-oz. bar	520
(Nestlé)	1 oz.	160
Chocolate Parfait (Pearson)	1 piece	30
Chocolate, Petite (Andes)	1 piece	26
Chuckles	1 oz.	92
Chunky (Nestlé):		
Regular	1 oz.	150
Deluxe nut	1 oz.	160
Clark Bar	1.5-oz. bar	201
Coffee Nip (Pearson)	1 piece	30
Coffioca Parfait (Pearson)	1 piece	30
Creme de Menthe (Andes)	1 piece	25
Crispy Bar (Clark)	1¼-oz. bar	187
Crows (Mason)	1 piece	11
Dutch Treat Bar (Clark)	1¹⁄₁₆-oz. bar	160
Eggs (Peter Paul Cadbury) creme	1 oz.	136
5th Avenue (Hershey's)	2.1-oz. bar	290
Fruit bears (Flavor Tree) assorted	½ of 2.1-oz. envelope	117
Fruit circus (Flavor Tree)	½ of 2.1-oz. envelope	117

Food and Description	Measure or Quantity	Calories
Fruit roll (Flavor Tree):		
Apple or cherry	¾-oz. roll	75
Strawberry	¾-oz. roll	74
Fudge (Nabisco) bar	1 piece	85
Goobers (Nestlé)	1 oz.	160
Good Stuff (Nab)	1.8-oz. piece	250
Halvah (Sahadi) original and marble	1 oz.	150
Hard (Jolly Rancher):		
All flavors except butterscotch	1 piece	23
Butterscotch	1 piece	25
Hollywood	1½-oz. bar	185
Jelly bean (*Chuckles*)	.5 oz.	55
Jelly rings, (*Chuckles*)	1 piece	37
Jujubes, (*Chuckles*)	.5 oz.	55
Ju Jus:		
Assorted	1 piece	7
Coins or raspberries	1 piece	15
Kisses (Hershey's)	1 piece	24
Kit Kat	1.6-oz. bar	250
Krackel Bar	1.55-oz. bar	230
Licorice:		
(Switzer) bars, bites or stix:		
Black	1 oz.	94
Cherry or strawberry	1 oz.	98
Chocolate	1 oz.	97
Twist:		
Black (American Licorice Co.)	1 piece	27
Black (Curtiss)	1 piece	27
Red (American Licorice Co.)	1 piece	33
Life Savers	1 piece	10
Lollipops (Life Savers)	1 pop	45
Mallo Cup (Boyer)	⁹⁄₁₆-oz. piece	54
Malted milk balls (Brach's)	1 piece	9
Mars Bar (M&M/Mars)	1.7-oz. bar	240
Marshmallow (Campfire)	1 oz.	111
Mary Jane (Miller):		
Small size	1.4 oz.	19
Large size	1½-oz. bar	110
Milk Duds (Clark)	¾-oz. box	89
Milk Shake (Hollywood Brands)	2.4-oz. bar	300
Milky Way (M&M/Mars)	2.24-oz. bar	290
Mint or peppermint:		
After dinner (Richardson):		
Jelly center	1 oz.	104
Regular	1 oz.	109
Canada Mint (Necco)	1 oz.	12
Chocolate-covered (Richardson)	1 oz.	106
Junior mint pattie (Nabisco)	1 piece	10
Mint Parfait (Andes)	1 piece	27

Food and Description	Measure or Quantity	Calories
Peppermint Pattie (Nabisco)	1 piece	55
York, pattie (Hershey's)	1.5-oz.	180
M&M's:		
Peanut	1.83-oz. pkg.	270
Plain	1.69-oz. pkg.	240
Mounds (Hershey's)	1.9-oz. serving	260
Mr. Goodbar (Hershey's)	1.75-oz. bar	290
Munch Bar (M&M/Mars)	1.42-oz. bar	220
My Buddy (Tom's)	1.8-oz. piece	250
Naturally Nut & Fruit Bar (Planters) almond/apricot	1 oz.	140
Necco Wafers, assorted	2.02-oz. roll	227
Nibs (Y&S)	1 oz.	100
Oh Henry! (Nestlé)	1 oz.	140
$100,000 Bar (Nestlé)	1.5-oz. bar	200
Orange slices (*Chuckles*)	1 oz.	110
Park Avenue (Tom's)	1.8-oz. bar	230
Payday (Hollywood Brands) regular	1.9-oz. bar	250
Peanut bar (Planters)	1.6 oz.	240
Peanut, chocolate-covered:		
(Curtiss)	1 piece	5
(Nabisco)	1 piece	11
Peanut butter cookie bar (M&M/Mars)	1¾-oz. serving	261
Peanut butter cup:		
(Boyer)	1.5-oz. pkg.	148
(Reese's)	.9-oz. cup	140
Peanut Butter Pals (Tom's)	1.3-oz. serving	200
Peanut crunch bar (Sahadi)	¾-oz. bar	110
Peanut Parfait (Andes)	1 piece	28
Peanut Plank (Tom's)	1.7-oz. piece	230
Peanut Roll (Tom's)	1.75-oz. piece	230
Powerhouse (Peter Paul Cadbury)	2 oz.	260
Raisin, chocolate-covered:		
(Nabisco)	1 piece	5
Raisinets (Nestlé)	1 oz.	120
Reese's Pieces (Hershey's)	1 piece	32
Reggie Bar	2-oz. bar	290
Rolo (Hershey's)	1 piece	34
Royals, mint chocolate (M&M/Mars)	1.52-oz. pkg.	212
Sesame Crunch (Sahadi)	¾-oz. bar	110
Skor (Hershey's)	1.4-oz. bar	220
Sky Bar (Necco)	1.5-oz. bar	198
Snickers	2-oz. bar	290
Solitaires (Hershey's)	½ of 3.2-oz. pkg.	260
Spearmint leaves (*Chuckles*)	1 oz.	110
Starburst (M&M/Mars)	1-oz. serving	120

Food and Description	Measure or Quantity	Calories
Sugar Babies (Nabisco)	1.6-oz. pkg.	180
Sugar Daddy (Nabisco) caramel sucker	1.4-oz. pop	150
Sugar Mama (Nabisco)	¾-oz. pop	90
Summit bar (M&M/Mars)	1 bar	115
Symphony (Hershey's)	1.4-oz. serving	220
Taffy, salt water (Brach's)	1 piece	31
3 Musketeers	.8-oz. bar	99
3 Musketeers	2.1-oz. bar	260
Ting-A-Ling (Andes)	1 piece	24
Tootsie Roll:		
Chocolate	.23-oz. midgee	26
Chocolate	¹⁄₁₆-oz. bar	72
Chocolate	1-oz. bar	115
Flavored	.6-oz. square	19
Pop, all flavors	.49-oz. pop	55
Pop drop, all flavors	4.7-gram piece	19
Twix Cookie bar (M&M/Mars)	1¾-oz. serving	246
Twizzlers	1 oz.	100
Whatchamacallit (Hershey's)	1.8-oz. bar	260
Wispa (Peter Paul Cadbury)	1 oz.	150
World Series Bar	1 oz.	128
Y & S Bites	1 oz.	100
Zagnut Bar (Clark)	.7-oz. bar	85
Zero (Hollywood Brands)	2-oz. bar	210
CANDY, DIETETIC:		
Caramel (Estee) chocolate or vanilla	1 piece	30
Carob bar, *Joan's Natural:*		
Coconut	3-oz. bar	516
Fruit & nut	3-oz. bar	559
Honey bran	3-oz. bar	487
Peanut	3-oz. bar	521
Chocolate or chocolate-flavored bar: (Estee):		
Coconut, fruit & nut or milk	.2-oz. square	30
Crunch	.2-oz. square	22
(Louis Sherry) coffee or orange-flavored	.2-oz. square	22
Estee-ets, with peanuts (Estee)	1 piece	7
Gum drops (Estee) any flavor	1 piece	6
Gummy Bears (Estee)	1 piece	7
Hard candy:		
(Estee) assorted fruit	1 piece	12
(Louis Sherry)	1 piece	12
Peanut brittle (Estee)	¼ oz.	35
Peanut butter cup (Estee)	1 cup	40
Raisins, chocolate-covered (Estee)	1 piece	3
CANDY APPLE COOLER DRINK, canned (Hi-C)	6 fl. oz.	94

Food and Description	Measure or Quantity	Calories
CANNELLONI, frozen:		
(Armour) *Dining Light*, cheese	9-oz. dinner	310
(Celentano)	12-oz. pkg.	350
(Stouffer's) beef & pork with mornay sauce, *Lean Cuisine*	9⅝-oz. pkg.	260
CANTALOUPE, cubed	½ cup (3 oz.)	24
CAPERS (Crosse & Blackwell)	1 tsp.	2
CAP'N CRUNCH, cereal (Quaker):		
Regular	¾ cup	121
Crunchberry	¾ cup	120
Peanut butter	¾ cup	127
CAPOCOLLO (Hormel)	1 oz.	80
CARAWAY SEED (French's)	1 tsp.	8
CARL'S JR. RESTAURANT:		
Bacon	2 strips (10 grams)	50
Cake, chocolate	3.2-oz. piece	380
California Roast Beef 'n Swiss Sandwich	7.2-oz. sandwich	360
Cheese:		
American	.6-oz. slice	63
Swiss	.6-oz. slice	57
Chicken sandwich:		
Charbroiler BBQ	6.3-oz. sandwich	320
Charbroiler Club	8.2-oz. sandwich	510
Cookie, chocolate chip	2¼-oz. piece	330
Danish	3.5-oz. piece	300
Eggs, scrambled	2.4-oz. serving	120
Fish sandwich, filet	7.9-oz. sandwich	550
French toast dips, excluding syrup	4.7-oz. serving	480
Hamburger:		
Plain:		
Famous Star	8.1-oz. serving	590
Happy Star	3.0-oz. serving	220
Old Time Star	5.9-oz. serving	400
Super Star	10.6-oz. serving	770
Cheeseburger, Western Bacon:		
Regular	7½-oz. serving	630
Double	10.4-oz. serving	890
Hot cake, with margarine, excluding syrup	5.5-oz. serving	360
Milk, 2% lowfat	10 fl. oz.	175
Muffins:		
Blueberry	3.5-oz. piece	256
Bran	4-oz. piece	220
English, with margarine	2-oz. piece	180
Onion rings	3.2-oz. order	310
Orange juice, small	8 fl. oz.	94

Food and Description	Measure or Quantity	Calories
Potato:		
Baked:		
Bacon & cheese	14.1-oz. serving	650
Broccoli & cheese	14-oz. serving	470
Cheese	14.2-oz. serving	550
Fiesta	15.2-oz. serving	550
Lite	9.8-oz. serving	250
Sour cream & chive	10.4-oz. serving	350
French fries	Regular order (6 oz.)	360
Hash brown nuggets	3-oz. serving	170
Salad dressing:		
Regular:		
Blue cheese	2-oz. serving	150
House	2-oz. serving	186
1000 Island	2-oz. serving	231
Dietetic, Italian	2-oz. serving	80
Sausage patty	1.5-oz. piece	190
Shake	1 regular size	353
Soft drink:		
Sweetened	1 regular size	243
Dietetic	1 regular size	2
Soup:		
Broccoli, cream of	1 serving	140
Chicken & noodle	1 serving	80
Clam chowder, Boston	1 serving	140
Vegetable, mixed	1 serving	70
Steak Sandwich, *Country Fried*		
Sunrise Sandwich:	7.2-oz. serving	610
Bacon	4.5-oz. serving	370
Sausage	6.1-oz. serving	500
Tea, iced	1 regular drink	2
Zucchini	4.3-oz. serving	300
CARNATION DO-IT-YOURSELF		
DIET PLAN	2 scoops	110
CARNATION INSTANT		
BREAKFAST:		
Bar:		
Chocolate chip	1 bar	200
Peanut butter crunch	1 bar	180
Packets, all flavors	1 packet	130
CARROT:		
Raw	5½" × 1" piece	21
Boiled, slices	½ cup	24
Canned, regular pack, solids & liq.:		
(Del Monte) sliced or whole	½ cup	30
(Larsen) *Freshlike*	½ cup	30
(Libby's)	½ cup	20

Food and Description	Measure or Quantity	Calories
Canned, dietetic pack, solids & liq., (S&W) *Nutradiet*, green label	½ cup	30
Frozen:		
(Birds Eye) deluxe	2.7 oz.	32
(Frosty Acres)	3.3 oz.	40
(Green Giant) cuts, in butter sauce	½ cup	80
(Larsen)	3.3 oz.	40
(Seabrook Farms)	⅓ pkg.	39
CASABA MELON	1-lb. melon	61
CASHEW BUTTER (Hain)	1 T.	95
CASHEW NUT:		
(Eagle Snacks) honey roast	1 oz.	170
(Fisher):		
Dry roasted	1 oz.	156
Honey, salted	1 oz.	150
Oil roasted	1 oz.	159
(Planters):		
Dry roasted	1 oz.	160
Honey roasted	1 oz.	170
Oil roasted	1 oz.	170
CATFISH, frozen (Mrs. Paul's) breaded & fried, fingers	4 oz.	250
CATSUP:		
Regular:		
(Del Monte)	1 T.	17
(Heinz)	1 T.	18
(Hunt's)	1 T.	15
(Smucker's)	1 T.	24
Dietetic or low calorie:		
(Del Monte) No Salt Added	1 T.	15
(Estee)	1 T.	6
(Featherweight)	1 T.	6
(Heinz) lite	1 T.	18
(Hunt's)	1 T.	20
(Weight Watchers)	1 T.	12
CAULIFLOWER:		
Raw or boiled buds	½ cup	14
Frozen:		
(Birds Eye) regular	3.3 oz.	23
(Frosty Acres)	3.3 oz.	25
(Green Giant):		
In cheese sauce:		
Regular	⅓ of 10-oz. pkg.	50
One Serving	5½-oz. serving	80
Polybag, cuts	2 oz.	12
(Larsen)	3.3 oz.	25
CAVATELLI, frozen (Celentano)	⅕ of 16-oz. pkg.	250

Food and Description	Measure or Quantity	Calories
CAVIAR:		
Pressed	1 oz.	90
Whole eggs	1 T.	42
CELERY:		
1 large outer stalk	8″ × 1½″ at root end	7
Diced or cut	½ cup	9
Frozen (Larsen)	3½ oz.	14
Salt (French's)	1 tsp.	12
Seed (French's)	1 tsp.	11
CEREAL (See brand name or specific type)		
CEREAL BAR (Kellogg's) *Smart Start*:		
Common Sense, oat bran with raspberry filling	1½-oz. bar	170
Nutri-Grain	1½-oz. bar	180
Rice Krispies, with almonds	1-oz. bar	130
CERTS	1 piece	6
CERVELAT (Hormel) Viking	1-oz. serving	90
CHABLIS WINE:		
(Almaden) light	3 fl. oz.	42
(Carlo Rossi)	3 fl. oz.	66
(Gallo) white or pink	3 fl. oz.	60
(Louis M. Martini)	3 fl. oz.	59
(Paul Masson):		
Regular	3 fl. oz.	71
Light	3 fl. oz.	45
CHAMPAGNE:		
(Bollinger)	3 fl. oz.	72
(Great Western):		
Regular	3 fl. oz.	71
Brut	3 fl. oz.	74
Pink	3 fl. oz.	81
(Taylor) dry	3 fl. oz.	78
CHARDONNAY WINE		
(Louis M. Martini)	3 fl. oz.	60
CHARLOTTE RUSSE, homemade recipe	4 oz.	324
CHEERIOS, cereal, regular, apple cinnamon, or honey & nut	1 oz.	110
CHEESE:		
American or cheddar:		
Cube, natural	1″ cube	68
(Borden)	1 oz.	110
(Churny) lite, cheddar, mild	1 oz.	80
(Dorman's):		
American:		
Lo-chol	1 oz.	90
Low sodium	1 oz.	110
Cheddar, light	1 oz.	80

Food and Description	Measure or Quantity	Calories
(Kraft):		
American Singles	1 oz.	90
Cheddar	1 oz.	110
Old English	1 oz.	110
(Land O'Lakes):		
Regular or with bacon	1 oz.	110
Chederella	1 oz.	100
Sharp or extra sharp	1 oz.	100
Laughing Cow, natural	1 oz.	110
(Polly-O) cheddar, shredded	1 oz.	110
(Sargento):		
Midget, regular or sharp	1 oz.	114
Shredded, non-dairy	1 oz.	90
Wispride	1 oz.	115
Blue:		
(Frigo)	1 oz.	100
(Kraft)	1 oz.	100
(Sargento) cold pack or crumbled	1 oz.	100
Bonbino, *Laughing Cow,* natural	1 oz.	103
Brick:		
(Land O'Lakes)	1 oz.	110
(Sargento) sliced	1 oz.	105
Brie (Sargento) *Danish Danko*	1 oz.	80
Burgercheese (Sargento)		
Danish Danko	1 oz.	106
Camembert (Sargento)		
Danish Danko	1 oz.	88
Colby:		
(Churny) lite	1 oz.	80
(Dorman's) *Lo-Chol*	1 oz.	100
(Kraft)	1 oz.	110
(Land O'Lakes)	1 oz.	110
(Pauly) low sodium	1 oz.	115
(Sargento) shredded or sliced	1 oz.	112
Cottage:		
Unflavored:		
(Bison):		
Regular	1 oz.	29
Dietetic	1 oz.	22
(Borden):		
Regular, 4% milkfat	½ cup	120
Lite-Line, 1.5% milkfat	½ cup	90
(Breakstone's) smooth & creamy	1 oz.	27
(Dairylea)	1 oz.	30
(Friendship)	1 oz.	30
(Johanna):		
Large or small curd	½ cup	120
No salt added	½ cup	90

Food and Description	Measure or Quantity	Calories
(Land O'Lakes)	1 oz.	30
(Light n' Lively)	1 oz.	20
(Sealtest)	1 oz.	30
(Weight Watchers) 1%	½ cup	90
Flavored (Friendship) pineapple	1 oz.	35
Cream, plain, unwhipped:		
(Frigo)	1 oz.	100
(Kraft) *Philadelphia Brand*:		
Regular	1 oz.	100
Light	1 oz.	60
Edam:		
(Churny) *May-Bud*	1 oz.	100
(House of Gold)	1 oz.	100
(Kaukauna)	1 oz.	100
(Kraft)	1 oz.	90
(Land O'Lakes)	1 oz.	100
Laughing Cow	1 oz.	100
Farmers:		
(Churny) *May-Bud*	1 oz.	90
Dutch Garden Brand	1 oz.	100
(Kaukauna)	1 oz.	100
(Sargento)	1 oz.	72
Wispride	1 oz.	100
Feta (Sargento) cups	1 oz.	76
Gjetost (Sargento) Norwegian	1 oz.	118
Gouda:		
(Churny) *May-Bud,* lite	1 oz.	81
(Kaukauna)	1 oz.	100
(Land O'Lakes)	1 oz.	100
Laughing Cow	1 oz.	110
(Sargento) baby, caraway or smoked	1 oz.	101
Wispride	1 oz.	100
Grated (Polly-O)	1 oz.	130
Gruyère, *Swiss Knight*	1 oz.	100
Havarti (Sargento):		
Creamy	1 oz.	90
Creamy, 60% mild	1 oz.	117
Hoop (Friendship) natural	1 oz.	21
Hot pepper (Sargento)	1 oz.	112
Jalapeño jack (Land O'Lakes)	1 oz.	90
Jarlsberg (Sargento) Norwegian	1 oz.	100
Kettle Moraine (Sargento)	1 oz.	100
Limburger (Sargento) natural	1 oz.	100
Monterey Jack:		
(Churny) lite	1 oz.	80
(Frigo)	1 oz.	100
(Kaukauna)	1 oz.	110
(Land O'Lakes)	1 oz.	110

Food and Description	Measure or Quantity	Calories
(Sargento) midget, Longhorn, shredded or sliced	1 oz.	106
Mozzarella:		
(Fisher) part skim milk	1 oz.	90
(Kraft)	1 oz.	80
(Polly-O):		
Fior di Latte	1 oz.	80
Part skim milk	1 oz.	80
Smoked	1 oz.	85
Whole milk:		
Regular or shredded	1 oz.	90
Old fashioned, regular	1 oz.	70
(Sargento):		
Bar, rounds, shredded regular or with spices, sliced for pizzas or square	1 oz.	79
Whole milk	1 oz.	100
Muenster:		
(Dorman's):		
Light	1 oz.	80
Lo-chol	1 oz.	100
Low sodium	1 oz.	110
(Kaukauna)	1 oz.	110
(Land O'Lakes)	1 oz.	100
(Sargento) red rind	1 oz.	104
Wispride	1 oz.	100
Nibblin Curds (Sargento)	1 oz.	114
Parmesan:		
(Frigo):		
Grated	1 T.	23
Whole	1 oz.	110
(Polly-O) grated	1 oz.	130
(Progresso) grated	1 T.	23
(Sargento):		
Grated	1 T.	27
Wedge	1 oz.	110
Pizza (Sargento) shredded or sliced	1 oz.	90
Pot (Sargento) regular, French onion or garlic	1 oz.	30
Provolone:		
(Dorman's) light	1 oz.	80
(Frigo)	1 oz.	90
(Land O'Lakes)	1 oz.	100
Laughing Cow:		
Cube	⅙ oz.	12
Wedge	¾ oz.	55
(Sargento) sliced	1 oz.	100
Ricotta:		
(Frigo) part skim milk	1 oz.	43

Food and Description	Measure or Quantity	Calories
(Polly-O):		
Lite	1 oz.	40
Part skim milk	1 oz.	45
Whole milk	1 oz.	50
(Sargento):		
Part skim milk	1 oz.	39
Whole milk	1 oz.	49
Romano:		
(Polly-O) grated	1 oz.	130
(Progresso) grated	1 T.	23
(Sargento) wedge	1 oz.	110
Roquefort, natural	1 oz.	104
Samsoe (Sargento) Danish	1 oz.	79
Scamorze (Frigo)	1 oz.	79
Semisoft, *Laughing Cow:*		
Babybel	1 oz.	90
Bonbel	1 oz.	100
Slim Jack (Dorman's)	1 oz.	80
Stirred curd (Frigo)	1 oz.	110
String (Sargento)	1 oz.	90
Swiss:		
(Churny) lite	1 oz.	90
(Dorman's) light	1 oz.	90
(Fisher) natural	1 oz.	100
(Frigo) domestic	1 oz.	100
(Sargento) domestic or Finland, sliced	1 oz.	107
Taco (Sargento) shredded	1 oz.	105
Washed curd (Frigo)	1 oz.	110
CHEESE FONDUE, *Swiss Knight*	1 oz.	110
CHEESE FOOD:		
American or cheddar:		
(Borden) *Lite Line*	1 oz.	50
(Fisher) *Ched-O-Mate* or *Sandwich-Mate*	1 oz.	90
Heart Beat (GFA)	⅔-oz. slice	35
(Weight Watchers) colored or white	1-oz. slice	50
Wispride:		
Regular	1 oz.	100
& port wine	1 oz.	100
Cheez-ola (Fisher)	1 oz.	90
Chef's Delight (Fisher)	1 oz.	70
Count Down (Pauly)	1 oz.	40
Cracker snack (Sargento)	1 oz.	90
Garlic & herbs, *Wispride*	1 oz.	90
Italian herb (Land O'Lakes)	1 oz.	90
Jalapeño (Borden) *Lite Line*	1 oz.	50
Loaf, *Count Down* (Pauly)	1 oz.	100

Food and Description	Measure or Quantity	Calories
Low sodium:		
(Borden) *Lite Line*	1 oz.	70
Heart Beat (GFA)	.7-oz. slice	35
Monterey Jack (Borden) *Lite Line*	1 oz.	50
Mun-chee (Pauly)	1 oz.	100
Neufchatel (Shedd's) Country Crock, any flavor	1 oz.	70
Onion (Land O'Lakes)	1 oz.	90
Pepperoni (Land O'Lakes)	1 oz.	90
Pimiento (Pauly)	.8-oz. slice	73
Pizza-Mate (Fisher)	1 oz.	90
Salami (Land O'Lakes)	1 oz.	90
Swiss:		
(Borden) *Lite Line*	1 oz.	50
(Kraft) reduced fat	1 oz.	90
CHEESE PUFFS, frozen (Durkee)	1 piece	59
CHEESE SPREAD:		
American or cheddar:		
(Fisher)	1 oz.	80
Laughing Cow	1 oz.	72
(Nabisco) *Easy Cheese*	1 tsp.	16
Blue, *Laughing Cow*	1 oz.	72
Cheese'n Bacon (Nabisco) *Easy Cheese*	1 tsp.	16
Golden velvet (Land O'Lakes)	1 oz.	80
Gruyère, *Laughing Cow, La Vache Que Rit,* reduced calorie	1 oz.	46
Provolone, *Laughing Cow*	1 oz.	72
Sharp (Pauly)	.8 oz.	77
Swiss, process (Pauly)	.8 oz.	76
Velveeta (Kraft)	1 oz.	80
CHEESE STRAW, frozen (Durkee)	1 piece	29
CHENIN BLANC WINE		
(Louis M. Martini)	3 fl. oz.	56
CHERRY, sweet:		
Fresh, with stems	½ cup (2.3 oz.)	41
Canned, regular pack (Del Monte) dark, solids & liq.	½ cup	50
Canned, dietetic, solids & liq.:		
(Diet Delight) with pits, water pack	½ cup	70
(Featherweight) dark, water pack	½ cup	60
(Thank You Brand)	½ cup	61
CHERRY, CANDIED	1 oz.	96
CHERRY DRINK:		
Canned:		
(Hi-C)	6 fl. oz.	100
(Lincoln) cherry berry	6 fl. oz.	100
(Smucker's) black	8 fl. oz.	130

Food and Description	Measure or Quantity	Calories
Squeezit (General Mills)	6¾-fl.-oz. container	110
Ssips (Johanna Farms)	8.45-fl.-oz. container	130
*Mix (Funny Face)	8 fl. oz.	88
CHERRY HEERING		
(Hiram Walker)	1 fl. oz.	80
CHERRY JELLY:		
Sweetened (Smucker's)	1 T.	54
Dietetic:		
(Dia-Mel)	1 T.	6
(Featherweight)	1 T.	16
(Smucker's)	⅜-oz. packet	4
CHERRY LIQUEUR (DeKuyper)	1 fl. oz.	75
CHERRY PRESERVES OR JAM:		
Sweetened (Smucker's)	1 T.	54
Dietetic (Estee)	1 T.	6
CHESTNUT, fresh, in shell	¼ lb.	220
CHEWING GUM:		
Sweetened:		
Bazooka, bubble	1 slice	18
Beechies	1 piece	6
Beech Nut; Beeman's Big Red; Black Jack; Clove; Doublemint; Freedent; Juicy Fruit, Spearmint (Wrigley's); *Teaberry*	1 stick	10
Bubble Yum	1 piece	25
Dentyne	1 piece	4
Extra (Wrigley's)	1 piece	8
Fruit Stripe, regular	1 piece	9
Hubba Bubba (Wrigley's)	1 piece	23
Dietetic:		
Bubble Yum	1 piece	20
Care Free, regular	1 piece	8
(Clark; *Care*Free*)	1 piece	7
(Estee) bubble or regular	1 piece	5
Extra (Wrigley's) cinnamon or spearmint	1 piece	8
(Featherweight) bubble or regular	1 piece	4
CHEX, cereal (Ralston Purina):		
Corn	1 cup (1 oz.)	110
Honey graham	⅔ cup	110
Rice	1⅛ cup (1 oz.)	110
Wheat	⅔ cup (1 oz.)	100
CHIANTI WINE:		
(Italian Swiss Colony)	3 fl. oz.	83
(Louis M. Martini)	3 fl. oz.	90
CHICKEN:		
Broiler, cooked, meat only	3 oz.	116
Fryer, fried, meat & skin	3 oz.	212

Food and Description	Measure or Quantity	Calories
Fryer, fried, meat only	3 oz.	178
Fryer, fried, 2½-lb. chicken (weighed with bone before cooking) will give you:		
Back	1 back	139
Breast	½ breast	160
Leg or drumstick	1 leg	87
Neck	1 neck	127
Rib	1 rib	41
Thigh	1 thigh	122
Wing	1 wing	82
Fried skin	1 oz.	119
Hen & cock:		
Stewed, dark meat only	3 oz.	176
Stewed, diced	½ cup	139
Stewed, light meat only	3 oz.	153
Stewed, meat & skin	3 oz.	269
Roaster, roasted, dark or light meat, without skin	3 oz.	156
CHICKEN À LA KING:		
Home recipe	1 cup	468
Canned (Swanson)	½ of 10½-oz. can	180
Frozen:		
(Armour) *Classics Lite*	11¼-oz. meal	290
(Banquet) *Cookin' Bag*	4-oz. pkg.	110
(Le Menu)	10¼-oz. dinner	320
(Stouffer's) with rice	9½-oz. pkg.	290
(Weight Watchers)	9-oz. pkg.	220
CHICKEN, BONED, canned:		
Regular:		
(Hormel) chunk, breast	6¾-oz. serving	350
(Swanson) chunk:		
Mixin' chicken	2½ oz.	130
White	2½ oz.	90
Low sodium (Featherweight)	2½ oz.	154
CHICKEN BOUILLON:		
Regular:		
(Herb-Ox):		
Cube	1 cube	6
Packet	1 packet	12
(Knorr)	1 cube	16
(Wyler's)	1 cube	8
Low sodium:		
(Featherweight)	1 tsp.	18
Lite-Line (Borden)	1 tsp.	12
CHICKEN CHUNKS, frozen (Country Pride):		
Regular	¼ of 12-oz. pkg.	240
Southern fried	¼ of 12-oz. pkg.	280

Food and Description	Measure or Quantity	Calories
CHICKEN, CREAMED, frozen (Stouffer's)	6½ oz.	300
CHICKEN DINNER OR ENTREE:		
Canned:		
(Hunt's) *Minute Gourmet Microwave Entree Maker:*		
Barbecued:		
Without chicken	3.1 oz.	150
*With chicken	6.8 oz.	320
Sweet & sour:		
Without chicken	4.1 oz.	130
*With chicken	7.8 oz.	300
(Swanson) & dumplings	7½ oz.	220
Frozen:		
(Armour):		
Classics Lite:		
Burgundy	10-oz. dinner	210
Sweet & sour	11-oz. dinner	240
Dining Lite, glazed	9-oz. meal	220
Dinner Classics:		
Glazed	10¾-oz. meal	300
Parmigiana	11¼-oz. meal	370
(Banquet):		
Cookin' Bag, & vegetable primavera	4-oz. serving	
Dinner:		
Regular:		
& dumplings	10-oz. dinner	430
Fried	10-oz. dinner	400
Extra Helping:		
Fried, all white meat	16-oz. dinner	570
Nuggets, with sweet & sour sauce	10-oz. dinner	650
Family Entree:		
& dumplings	¼ of 28-oz. pkg.	280
& vegetable primavera	¼ of 28-oz. pkg.	140
Platter:		
Boneless, pattie	7½-oz. meal	380
Fried, all white meat, hot 'n spicy	9-oz. meal	430
(Celentano):		
Parmigiana	9-oz. meal	400
Primavera	11½-oz. pkg.	260
(Chun King) & walnuts, crunchy	13-oz. meal	310
(Healthy Choice):		
A l'orange	9½-oz. meal	260
Herb roasted	11-oz. meal	260
Mesquite	10½-oz. meal	310
Sweet & sour	11½-oz. meal	280

Food and Description	Measure or Quantity	Calories
(Kid Cuisine):		
Fried	7¼-oz. meal	420
Nuggets	6¼-oz. meal	400
(La Choy) Fresh and Lite:		
Almond with rice and vegetables	9¾-oz. meal	270
Oriental, spicy	9¾-oz. meal	270
(Le Menu) sweet & sour	11¼-oz. dinner	450
(Morton):		
Regular:		
Boneless	11-oz. dinner	329
Fried	11-oz. pkg.	431
Light, boneless	11-oz. dinner	250
(Stouffer's):		
Regular:		
Cashew in sauce, with rice	9½-oz. meal	380
Divan	8½-oz. meal	320
Lean Cuisine:		
Glazed with vegetable rice	8½-oz. serving	270
& vegetables with vermicelli	12¾-oz. serving	260
Right Course:		
Italiano, with fettucini & vegetables	9⅝-oz. meal	280
Sesame	10-oz. meal	320
Tenderloin, in barbecue sauce with rice pilaf	8¾-oz. meal	270
(Swanson):		
Regular:		
& dumplings	7½-oz. meal	220
Fried, 4-compartment:		
Barbecue flavor	9¼-oz. dinner	560
Dark meat	10¼-oz. dinner	610
Hungry Man:		
Boneless	17½-oz. dinner	670
Parmigiana	20-oz. dinner	810
(Tyson):		
À l'orange	9½-oz. meal	300
Français	9½-oz. meal	290
Parmigiana	11¼-oz. meal	380
(Weight Watchers):		
Cordon bleu, breaded	8-oz. meal	230
Fettucini	8¼-oz. meal	290
Patty, southern fried	6½-oz. meal	340
Sweet & sour tenders	10.2-oz. meal	240
CHICKEN, FRIED, frozen:		
(Banquet):		
Assorted	32-oz. pkg.	1,650
Breast portion	11½-oz. pkg.	440
Hot 'n spicy, thigh & drumstick	12½-oz. meal	500

Food and Description	Measure or Quantity	Calories
(County Pride) southern fried, patties	3 oz.	232
(Swanson) *Plump & Juicy:*		
Assorted	3¼-oz. serving	270
Breast portions	4½-oz. serving	350
Nibbles	3¼-oz. serving	300
Take-out style	3¼-oz. serving	270
*CHICKEN HELPER (General Mills):		
& dumplings	⅕ pkg.	530
& mushrooms	⅕ pkg.	470
Teriyaki	⅕ pkg.	480
CHICKEN & NOODLES, frozen:		
(Armour):		
Dining Lite	9-oz. meal	240
Dinner Classics	11-oz. meal	230
(Stouffer's):		
Escalloped	5¾-oz. serving	252
Paprikash	10½-oz. serving	391
CHICKEN NUGGETS, frozen (See also CHICKEN DINNER OR ENTREE, HOT BITES, etc.):		
(Country Pride)	¼ of 12-oz. pkg.	250
(Empire Kosher)	¼ of 12-oz. pkg.	177
CHICKEN, PACKAGED:		
(Carl Buddig) smoked	1 oz.	60
(Louis Rich) breast, oven roasted	1-oz. slice	40
(Weaver):		
Bologna	1 slice	44
Breast, oven roasted	1 slice	25
Roll	1 slice	26
CHICKEN PATTY, frozen:		
(Country Pride):		
Regular	¼ of 12-oz. pkg.	250
Southern fried	¼ of 12-oz. pkg.	240
(Empire Kosher Poultry)	¼ of 12-oz. pkg.	198
CHICKEN PIE, frozen:		
(Banquet) regular	8-oz. pie	550
(Empire Kosher)	8-oz. pie	463
(Stouffer's)	10-oz. pie	530
(Swanson) regular	8-oz. pie	420
CHICKEN PUFF, frozen (Durkee)	½-oz. piece	49
CHICKEN SALAD (Carnation)	¼ of 7½-oz. can	94
CHICKEN SOUP (See SOUP, Chicken)		
CHICKEN SPREAD:		
(Hormel) regular	1 oz.	60
(Underwood) chunky	½ of 4¾-oz. can	63
CHICKEN STEW, canned:		

Food and Description	Measure or Quantity	Calories
Regular:		
(Libby's) with dumplings	8 oz.	194
(Swanson)	7⅜ oz.	170
Dietetic (Dia-Mel)	8-oz. serving	150
CHICKEN STICKS, frozen (Country Pride)	3 oz.	233
CHICKEN STOCK BASE (French's)	1 tsp.	8
CHICK-FIL-A:		
Brownie, fudge, with nuts	2.8-oz. piece	369
Chicken, no bun	3.6-oz. serving	219
Chicken nuggets, 8-pack	4 oz.	287
Chicken salad:		
Regular:		
Cup	3.4-oz. serving	309
Plate	11.8-oz. serving	475
Chargrilled, golden	16.4-oz. serving	126
Sandwich, Chargrilled	5½-oz. serving	258
Chicken sandwich, with bun:		
Regular	5¾-oz. serving	360
Deluxe Chargrilled, with lettuce & tomato	7.15-oz. serving	266
Coleslaw	3.7-oz. cup	175
Icedream	4½-oz. serving	135
Pie, lemon	4.1-oz. piece	329
Potato, *Waffle Potato Fries*	3-oz. serving	270
Potato salad	3.8-oz. serving	198
Salad, tossed:		
Plain	4½-oz. serving	21
With dressing:		
Honey french	6-oz. serving	246
Italian, light	6-oz. serving	46
1000 Island	6-oz. serving	231
Soup, hearty breast of chicken, small	8½-oz. serving	152
CHICK'N QUICK, frozen (Tyson):		
Breast fillet	3 oz.	190
Breast pattie	3 oz.	240
Chick'N Cheddar	3 oz.	260
Cordon bleu	5 oz.	310
Kiev	5 oz.	430
CHICK PEA OR GARBANZO, canned, solids & liq.:		
(Allen's; Goya)	½ cup	110
(Progresso)	½ cup	120
CHILI OR CHILI CON CARNE:		
Canned, regular pack:		
Beans only:		
(Comstock)	½ cup	140
(Hormel)	5 oz.	130
(Hunt's)	1 cup	200

Food and Description	Measure or Quantity	Calories
(Van Camp) Mexican style	1 cup	250
With beans:		
(Gebhardt) hot	½ of 15-oz. can	470
(Hormel) regular or hot	7½-oz. serving	310
Just Rite (Hunt's) hot	4 oz.	195
(Libby's)	7½-oz. serving	270
(Old El Paso)	1 cup	217
(Swanson)	7¾-oz. serving	310
Without beans:		
(Gebhardt)	½ of 15-oz. can	410
(Hormel) regular or hot	7½-oz. serving	370
Just Rite (Hunt's)	4-oz. serving	180
(Libby's)	7½ oz.	390
Canned, dietetic pack:		
(Estee) with beans	8-oz. serving	370
(Featherweight) with beans	7½ oz.	270
Frozen (Stouffer's):		
Regular, with beans	8¾-oz. meal	260
Right Choice, vegetarian	9¾-oz. meal	280
*Mix, *Manwich, Chili Fixins*	8 oz.	290
CHILI SAUCE:		
(Del Monte)	¼ cup (2 oz.)	70
(El Molino) green, mild	1 T.	5
(Heinz)	1 T.	17
(La Victoria)	1 T.	3
(Ortega) green, medium	1 oz.	7
(Featherweight) dietetic	1 T.	8
CHILI SEASONING MIX:		
*(Durkee)	1 cup	465
(French's) *Chili-O*, plain	1¾-oz. pkg.	150
(Lawry's)	1.6-oz. pkg.	143
(McCormick)	1.2-oz. pkg.	106
CHIMICHANGA, frozen:		
Marquez (Fred's Frozen Foods), beef, shredded	5-oz. serving	351
(Old El Paso):		
Regular, chicken	1 piece	360
Dinner, festive, beef	11-oz. dinner	540
Entree, bean & cheese	1 piece	350
CHOCOLATE, BAKING:		
(Baker's):		
Milk, chips	1 oz.	152
Semi-sweet:		
Chocolate flavored:		
Chips	¼ cup	212
Square	1 oz.	150
Real	¼ cup	224
Sweetened, *German's*:		
Chips	¼ cup	230

Food and Description	Measure or Quantity	Calories
Square	1 oz.	158
(Hershey's):		
Bitter or unsweetened	1 oz.	190
Sweetened:		
Milk:		
Chips:		
Regular	1 oz.	150
Vanilla	1 oz.	160
Chunks	1 oz.	160
Semi-sweet:		
Bar or chunks	1 oz.	140
Chips	1 oz.	147
(Nestlé):		
Bitter or unsweetened, *Choco-bake*	1-oz. packet	180
Sweet or semi-sweet, morsels	1 oz.	150
CHOCOLATE ICE CREAM		
(See ICE CREAM, Chocolate)		
CHOCOLATE SYRUP		
(See SYRUP, Chocolate)		
CHOP SUEY, frozen (Stouffer's)		
beef with rice	12-oz. pkg.	340
*CHOP SUEY SEASONING MIX		
(Durkee)	1¾ cups	557
CHOWDER (See SOUP, Chowder)		
CHOW MEIN:		
Canned:		
(Chun King) Divider-Pak:		
Beef	¼ pkg.	91
Chicken	½ of 24-oz. pkg.	110
Shrimp	¼ pkg.	91
(Hormel) pork, *Short Orders*	7½-oz. can	140
(La Choy):		
Regular:		
Beef	¾ cup	60
Chicken	¾ cup	70
Shrimp	¾ cup	45
*Bi-pack:		
Beef	¾ cup	70
Beef pepper oriental, chicken or shrimp	¾ cup	80
Vegetable	¾ cup	50
Frozen:		
(Armour) *Dining Lite,* chicken & rice	9-oz. dinner	180
(Chun King) chicken	13-oz. entree	370
(Empire Kosher)	½ of 15-oz. pkg.	97
(Healthy Choice)	8½-oz. meal	220
(La Choy):		
Chicken	12-oz. dinner	260

Food and Description	Measure or Quantity	Calories
Shrimp	12-oz. dinner	220
(Stouffer's) *Lean Cuisine,* with rice	11¼-oz. serving	250
CHOW MEIN SEASONING MIX (Kikkoman)	1⅛-oz. pkg.	98
CHURCH'S FRIED CHICKEN:		
Chicken, fried:		
Breast	4.3-oz. piece	278
Leg	2.9-oz. piece	147
Thigh	4.2-oz. piece	306
Wing-breast	4.8-oz. piece	303
Corn, with butter oil	1 ear	237
French fried potatoes	1 regular order	138
CHUTNEY (Major Grey's)	1 T.	53
CINNAMON, GROUND (French's)	1 tsp.	6
CINNAMON TOAST CRUNCH, cereal (General Mills)	¾ cup	120
CITRUS BERRY BLEND, mix, dietetic (Sunkist)	8 fl. oz.	6
CITRUS COOLER DRINK, canned:		
(Five Alive)	6 fl. oz.	87
(Hi-C)	6 fl. oz.	95
CLAM:		
Raw, all kinds, meat only	1 cup (8 oz.)	186
Raw, soft, meat & liq.	1 lb. (weighed in shell)	142
Canned (Doxsee):		
Chopped, minced or whole:		
Solids & liquid	½ cup	97
Drained solids	½ cup	58
Canned (Gorton's) minced, meat only	1 can	140
Frozen:		
(Gorton's) strips, crunchy	3½ oz.	330
(Howard Johnson's)	5-oz. pkg.	395
(Mrs. Paul's) fried, light	2½-oz. serving	230
CLAMATO COCKTAIL (Mott's)	6 fl. oz.	96
CLAM JUICE (Snow)	½ cup	15
CLARET WINE:		
(Gold Seal)	3 fl. oz.	82
(Taylor) 12.5% alcohol	3 fl. oz.	72
CLORETS, gum or mint	1 piece	6
CLUSTERS, cereal (General Mills)	½ cup	110
COBBLER, frozen (Pet-Ritz):		
Apple or strawberry	⅙ of 26-oz. pkg.	290
Blackberry	⅙ of 26-oz. pkg.	270
Cherry	⅙ of 26-oz. pkg.	280
COCKTAIL (See individual listings		

Food and Description	Measure or Quantity	Calories
such as **DAIQUIRI, PIÑA COLADA**, etc.)		
COCOA:		
Dry, unsweetened:		
(Hershey's) regular	1 T.	22
(Sultana)	1 T.	30
Mix, regular:		
(Alba '66) instant, all flavors	1 envelope	60
(Carnation) all flavors	1-oz. pkg.	110
(Hershey's) instant	3 T.	81
(Ovaltine) hot 'n rich	1 oz.	120
Swiss Miss, regular or with mini marshmallows	6 fl. oz.	110
Mix, dietetic:		
(Carnation):		
70 Calorie	¾-oz. packet	70
*Sugar free	6 fl. oz.	50
Swiss Miss, instant, lite	1 envelope	70
(Weight Watchers)	1 envelope	60
COCOA KRISPIES, cereal		
(Kellogg's)	¾ cup (1 oz.)	110
COCOA PUFFS, cereal		
(General Mills)	1 cup (1 oz.)	110
COCONUT:		
Fresh, meat only	2″ × 2″ × ½″ piece	156
Grated or shredded, loosely packed	½ cup	225
Dried:		
(Baker's):		
Angel Flake	⅓ cup	118
Cookie	⅓ cup	186
Premium shred	⅓ cup	138
(Durkee) shredded	¼ cup	69
COCONUT, CREAM OF, canned:		
(Coco Lopez)	1 T.	60
(Holland House)	1 oz.	81
COCO WHEATS, cereal (Little Crow)	1 T.	43
COD:		
Broiled	3 oz.	145
Frozen:		
(Frionor) *Norway Gourmet*	4-oz. fillet	70
(Van de Kamp's) *Today's Catch*	4-oz.	80
COD DINNER OR ENTREE, frozen:		
(Armour) *Dinner Classics,* almondine	12-oz. dinner	360
(Frionor) *Norway Gourmet*, with dill sauce	4½-oz. fillet	80
COD LIVER OIL (Hain)	1 T.	120

Food and Description	Measure or Quantity	Calories
COFFEE:		
Regular:		
*Max-Pax; Maxwell House Electra Perk; Yuban, Yuban Electra Matic	6 fl. oz.	2
*Mellow Roast	6 fl.oz.	8
Decaffeinated:		
*Brim, regular or electric perk	6 fl. oz.	2
*Sanka, regular or electric perk	6 fl. oz.	2
*Instant:		
Regular:		
Maxwell House; Taster's Choice	6 fl. oz.	4
Mellow Roast	6 fl. oz.	8
Sunrise	6 fl. oz.	6
Decaffeinated:		
*Brim, freeze-dried; Decafé; Nescafé	6 fl. oz.	4
*Mix (General Foods)		
International Coffee:		
Café Amaretto, Café Français	6 fl. oz.	59
Café Vienna, Orange Cappuccino	6 fl. oz.	65
Suisse Mocha	6 fl. oz.	58
COFFEE CAKE (See CAKE, Coffee)		
COFFEE LIQUEUR (DeKuyper)	1½ fl. oz.	140
COFFEE SOUTHERN	1 fl. oz.	79
COGNAC (See DISTILLED LIQUOR)		
COLA SOFT DRINK (See SOFT DRINK, Cola)		
COLD DUCK WINE (Great Western) pink	3 fl. oz.	92
COLESLAW, solids & liq., made with mayonnaise-type salad dressing	1 cup	119
***COLESLAW MIX** (Libby's) Super Slaw	½ cup	240
COLLARDS:		
Leaves, cooked	⅓ pkg.	31
Canned (Allen's) chopped, solids & liq.	½ cup	25
Frozen:		
(Birds Eye) chopped	⅓ pkg.	30
(McKenzie) chopped	⅓ pkg.	25
(Southland) chopped	⅕ of 16-oz. pkg.	25
COMPLETE CEREAL (Elam's)	1 oz.	109
CONCORD WINE:		
(Gold Seal)	3 fl. oz.	125
(Pleasant Valley) red	3 fl. oz.	90

Food and Description	Measure or Quantity	Calories
COOKIE, REGULAR:		
Almond Supreme (Pepperidge Farm)	1 piece	70
Angelica Goodies (Stella D'Oro)	1 piece	110
Angel Wings (Stella D'Oro)	1 piece	70
Anginetti (Stella D'Oro)	1 piece	30
Animal:		
(Dixie Belle)	1 piece	8
(FFV)	1 piece	14
(Nabisco) *Barnum's Animals*	1 piece	12
(Sunshine)	1 piece	8
(Tom's)	½ oz.	62
Anisette sponge (Stella D'Oro)	1 piece	50
Anisette toast (Stella D'Oro):		
Regular	1 piece	50
Jumbo	1 piece	110
Apple N' Raisin (Archway)	1 cookie	120
Apricot Raspberry (Pepperidge Farm)	1 piece	50
Assortment:		
(Nabisco) *Mayfair:*		
Crown creme sandwich	1 piece	53
Fancy shortbread biscuit	1 piece	22
Filigree creme sandwich	1 piece	60
Mayfair creme sandwich	1 piece	65
Tea rose creme	1 piece	53
(Pepperidge Farm):		
Butter	1 piece	55
Champagne	1 piece	32
Chocolate lace & Pirouette	1 piece	37
Seville	1 piece	55
Southport	1 piece	75
(Stella D'Oro) hostess or *Lady Stella*	1 piece	40
Blueberry (Pepperidge Farm)	1 piece	57
Blueberry Newtons (Nabisco)	1 piece	73
Bordeaux (Pepperidge Farm)	1 piece	33
Breakfast treats (Stella D'Oro)	1 piece	100
Brown edge wafer (Nabisco)	1 piece	28
Brownie:		
(Hostess)	1.25-oz. piece	157
(Nabisco) *Almost Home*	1¼-oz. piece	160
(Pepperidge Farm) chocolate nut	.4-oz. piece	57
Brussels (Pepperidge Farm)	1 piece	53
Brussels Mint (Pepperidge Farm)	1 piece	67
Butter (Sunshine)	1 piece	30
Cappuccino (Pepperidge Farm)	1 piece	53
Caramel Patties (FFV)	1 piece	75

Food and Description	Measure or Quantity	Calories
Castelets (Stella D'Oro)	1 piece	70
Chessman (Pepperidge Farm)	1 piece	43
Chocolate & chocolate-covered:		
(Keebler) stripes	1 piece	50
(Nabisco):		
Pinwheel, cake	1 piece	130
Snap	1 piece	19
(Sunshine) nuggets	1 piece	23
Chocolate chip:		
(Keebler) Rich 'n Chips	1 piece	80
(Nabisco):		
Almost Home	1 piece	65
Chips Ahoy!:		
Regular	1 piece	47
Chewy	1 piece	65
Snaps	1 piece	22
(Pepperidge Farm):		
Regular	1 piece	50
Chocolate	1 piece	53
Mocha	1 piece	40
(Sunshine):		
Chip-A-Roos	1 piece	60
Chippy Chews	1 piece	50
(Tom's)	1.7-oz. serving	230
Coconut fudge (FFV)	1 piece	80
Como Delights (Stella D'Oro)	1 piece	150
Date Nut Granola (Pepperidge Farm)	1 piece	53
Dinosaurs (FFV)	1 oz.	130
Dutch apple bar (Stella D'Oro)	1 piece	110
Dutch cocoa (Archway)	1 piece	110
Egg biscuit (Stella D'Oro):		
Regular	1 piece	80
Roman	1 piece	140
Egg jumbo (Stella D'Oro)	1 piece	50
Fig bar:		
(FFV)	1 piece	70
(Nabisco) *Fig Newtons*	1 piece	50
(Sunshine) Chewies	1 piece	50
(Tom's)	1.8-oz. serving	170
Fruit Stick (Nabisco) *Almost Home*	1 piece	70
Fudge (Stella D'Oro) swiss	1 piece	70
Gingerman (Pepperidge Farm)	1 piece	57
Ginger snap:		
(Archway)	1 piece	25
(FFV)	1 oz.	130
(Nabisco)	1 piece	30
(Sunshine)	1 piece	20
Golden bars (Stella D'Oro)	1 piece	110
Golden Fruit Raisin (Sunshine)	1 piece	70

Food and Description	Measure or Quantity	Calories
Hazelnut (Pepperidge Farm)	1 piece	57
Jelly tarts (FFV)	1 piece	60
Ladyfinger	3¼" × 1⅜" × 1⅛"	40
Lido (Pepperidge Farm)	1 piece	95
Macaroon, coconut (Nabisco)	1 piece	95
Mallow Puffs (Sunshine)	1 piece	70
Margherite (Stella D'Oro)	1 piece	70
Marshmallow:		
(Nabisco):		
Mallomars	1 piece	65
Puffs, cocoa covered	1 piece	120
Sandwich	1 piece	30
Twirls cakes	1 piece	130
(Planters) banana pie	1 oz.	127
Milano (Pepperidge Farm)	1 piece	60
Mint Milano (Pepperidge Farm)	1 piece	76
Molasses:		
(Archway)	1 piece	100
(Nabisco) *Pantry*	1 piece	65
Molasses Crisp (Pepperidge Farm)	1 piece	33
Nilla wafer (Nabisco)	1 piece	19
Oatmeal:		
(Archway):		
Regular	1 piece	110
Date filled	1 piece	100
(FFV) bar	1 piece	70
(Keebler) old fashioned	1 piece	80
(Nabisco) *Bakers Bonus*	1 piece	65
(Pepperidge Farm):		
Irish	1 piece	47
Raisin	1 piece	57
(Sunshine) Country	1 piece	60
Orange Milano (Pepperidge Farm)	1 piece	76
Orbits (Sunshine)	1 piece	15
Peach apricot bar (FFV)	1 piece	70
Peanut & peanut butter (Nabisco):		
Almost Home	1 piece	70
Nutter Butter, sandwich	1 piece	70
Pecan Sandies (Keebler)	1 piece	80
Pfenernusse (Stella D'Oro)	1 piece	40
Raisin:		
(Nabisco) *Almost Home:*		
Fudge chocolate chip	1 piece	65
Iced applesauce	1 piece	70
(Pepperidge Farm) bran	1 piece	53
Raisin bran (Pepperidge Farm) *Kitchen Hearth*	1 piece	53
Raspberry filled (Archway)	1 cookie	105
Rocky road (Archway)	1 cookie	130

Food and Description	Measure or Quantity	Calories
Royal Dainty (FFV)	1 piece	60
Sandwich:		
(FFV) mint	1 piece	80
(Keebler):		
Fudge creme	1 piece	60
Pitter Patter	1 piece	90
(Nabisco):		
Baronet	1 piece	47
Gaity	1 piece	50
Giggles	1 piece	70
I Screams	1 piece	75
Oreo, regular	1 piece	47
Almost Home	1 piece	140
(Sunshine):		
Regular, *Hydrox*	1 piece	50
Chips 'n Middles	1 piece	70
Tru Blu	1 piece	80
Sesame (Stella D'Oro) regina	1 piece	50
Shortbread or shortcake:		
(FFV) country	1 piece	70
(Nabisco):		
Lorna Doone	1 piece	35
Pecan	1 piece	75
(Pepperidge Farm)	1 piece	75
Social Tea, biscuit (Nabisco)	1 piece	22
Sprinkles (Sunshine)	1 piece	70
Sugar cookie (Nabisco) rings, *Bakers Bonus*	1 piece	65
Sugar wafer:		
(Dutch Twin) any flavor	1 piece	36
(Nabisco) *Biscos*	1 piece	19
(Sunshine)	1 piece	45
Tahiti (Pepperidge Farm)	1 piece	85
Toy (Sunshine)	1 piece	12
Vanilla wafer (FFV)	1 piece	130
Waffle creme (Dutch Twin)	1 piece	45
COOKIE, DIETETIC:		
Apple pastry (Stella D'Oro)	1 piece	90
Chocolate chip (Estee)	1 piece	30
Coconut:		
(Estee)	1 piece	30
(Stella D'Oro)	1 piece	50
Egg biscuit (Stella D'Oro)	1 piece	40
Fruit & honey (Entenmann's)	1 piece	40
Fudge (Estee))	1 piece	30
Kichel (Stella D'Oro)	1 piece	8
Oatmeal raisin:		
(Entenmann's)	1 piece	40

Food and Description	Measure or Quantity	Calories
(Estee)	1 piece	30
Prune pastry (Stella D'Oro)	1 piece	90
Sandwich (Estee) original	1 piece	45
Sesame (Stella D'Oro) regina	1 piece	40
Wafer, creme filled (Estee)	1 piece	30
COOKIE CRISP, cereal, any flavor (Ralston Purina)	1 cup	110
*COOKIE DOUGH:		
Refrigerated (Pillsbury):		
Brownie, microwave, with chocolate chips	1 piece	180
Oatmeal raisin or peanut butter	1 cookie	70
Frozen (Rich's):		
Chocolate chip	1 cookie	138
Oatmeal	1 cookie	125
COOKIE MIX:		
Regular:		
Brownie:		
*(Betty Crocker):		
Chocolate chip	¹⁄₂₄ of pan	130
Frosted	¹⁄₂₄ of pan	160
Fudge, family size	¹⁄₂₄ of pan	130
Walnut	¹⁄₂₄ of pan	140
(Duncan Hines):		
Chewy	¹⁄₂₄ pkg.	98
Fudge, original	¹⁄₂₄ pkg.	122
Peanut butter	¹⁄₂₄ pkg.	120
Truffle	¹⁄₁₆ pkg.	200
*(Gold Medal) fudge	¹⁄₁₆ pkg.	100
*(Pillsbury) fudge:		
Regular	2″ sq. (¹⁄₁₆ pkg.)	150
Microwave	⅑ of pkg.	190
Ultimate, rocky road	2″ sq. (¹⁄₁₆ of pkg.)	170
Chocolate chip:		
*(Betty Crocker) *Big Batch*	1 cookie	60
*(Duncan Hines)	¹⁄₃₆ pkg.	73
*(Quaker)	1 cookie	75
*Fudge chip (Quaker)	1 cookie	75
*Macaroon, coconut (Betty Crocker)	¹⁄₂₄ pkg.	80
Oatmeal (Duncan Hines) raisin	¹⁄₃₆ pkg.	68
Peanut butter (Duncan Hines)	¹⁄₃₆ pkg.	68
Sugar		
Dietetic (Estee) brownie	2″ × 2″ sq. cookie	45
COOKING SPRAY:		
Mazola No Stick	2½-second spray	6
(Weight Watchers)	2½-second spray	5
Wesson Lite	2-second spray	<1

Food and Description	Measure or Quantity	Calories
CORN:		
Fresh, on the cob, boiled	5″ × 1¾″ ear	70
Canned, regular pack, solids & liq.:		
(Allen's) whole kernel	½ cup	80
(Comstock) whole kernel	½ cup	90
(Del Monte):		
Cream style, golden	½ cup	95
Whole kernel	½ cup	100
(Green Giant):		
Cream style	4¼ oz.	100
Whole kernel, golden	4¼ oz.	80
Whole kernel, *Mexicorn*	3½ oz.	80
(Larsen) *Freshlike,* whole kernel, vacuum pack	½ cup	100
(Libby's) cream style	½ cup	100
(Stokely-Van Camp):		
Cream style	½ cup	105
Whole kernel, solids & liq.	½ cup	74
Canned, dietetic pack, solids & liq.:		
(Diet Delight)	½ cup	60
(Green Giant)	½ cup	80
(Larsen) *Fresh-Lite*	½ cup	80
(S&W) *Nutradiet,* whole kernel, green label	½ cup	80
Frozen:		
(Birds Eye):		
On the cob:		
Regular	4.4-oz. ear	120
Little Ears	4.6-oz. ear	126
With butter sauce	⅓ pkg.	85
(Frosty Acres):		
On the cob	1 whole ear	120
Kernels	3.3 oz.	80
(Green Giant):		
On the cob, regular:		
Nibbler	1 ear	60
Niblet ear	1 ear	120
Whole kernel, butter sauce, golden	4 oz.	100
Whole kernel, *Niblets,* golden, polybag	⅓ pkg.	80
(Larsen):		
On the cob	3″ piece (2.2 oz.)	60
Kernels	3.3 oz.	80
(Ore-Ida) cob corn	5.3-oz. ear	160
(Seabrook Farms):		
On the cob	5″ ear	140
Whole kernel	⅓ pkg.	97

Food and Description	Measure or Quantity	Calories
CORNBREAD:		
Home recipe:		
Corn pone	4 oz.	231
Spoon bread	4 oz.	221
*Mix:		
(Aunt Jemima)	⅙ pkg.	220
Gold Medal (General Mills)	⅙ pkg.	150
(Pillsbury) *Ballard*	⅛ of recipe	140
***CORN DOGS,** frozen		
(Hormel)	1 piece	220
CORNED BEEF:		
Cooked, boneless, medium fat	4-oz. serving	422
Canned, regular pack:		
Dinty Moore (Hormel)	2-oz. serving	130
(Libby's)	⅓ of 7-oz. can	160
Canned, dietetic (Featherweight)		
loaf	2½-oz. serving	90
Packaged (Carl Buddig) sliced	1-oz. slice	40
CORNED BEEF HASH, canned:		
(Libby's)	⅓ of 24-oz. can	420
Mary Kitchen (Hormel)	7½-oz. serving	360
CORNED BEEF HASH DINNER,		
frozen (Banquet)	10-oz. dinner	372
CORNED BEEF SPREAD		
(Underwood)	½ of 4½-oz. can	120
CORN FLAKE CRUMBS		
(Kellogg's)	¼ cup	100
CORN FLAKES, cereal:		
(General Mills) *Country*	1 cup (1 oz.)	110
(Kellogg's) regular	1 cup (1 oz.)	110
(Malt-O-Meal) sugar-coated	¾ cup	109
(Ralston Purina) regular	1 cup	110
CORN MEAL:		
Bolted (Aunt Jemima/Quaker)	3 T.	102
Degermed	¼ cup	125
Mix, bolted (Aunt Jemima) white	1 cup	392
***CORN POPS,** cereal		
(Kellogg's)	1 cup	110
CORN PUREE (Larsen)	½ cup	100
CORNSTARCH (Argo; Kingsford's; Duryea)	1 tsp.	10
CORN SYRUP (See SYRUP, Corn)		
COUGH DROP:		
(Beech-Nut)	1 drop	10
(Pine Bros.)	1 drop	10
***COUNT CHOCULA,** cereal		
(General Mills)	1 cup (1 oz.)	110
CRAB:		
Fresh, steamed:		
Whole	½ lb.	101

Food and Description	Measure or Quantity	Calories
Meat only	4 oz.	105
Canned, drained	4 oz.	115
Frozen (Wakefield's)	4 oz.	96
CRAB, IMITATION (Louis Kemp)		
Crab Delights, chunks, flakes or legs	2 oz.	60
CRAB APPLE, flesh only	¼ lb.	71
CRAB APPLE JELLY (Smucker's)	1 T.	54
CRAB, DEVILED, frozen		
(Mrs. Paul's) breaded & fried,		
regular	½ of 6-oz. pkg.	170
CRAB IMPERIAL, home recipe	1 cup	323
CRACKERS, PUFFS & CHIPS:		
Animal (FFV)	1 oz.	130
Arrowroot biscuit (Nabisco)	1 piece	22
Bacon-flavored thins (Nabisco)	1 piece	10
Bacon Nips	1 oz.	147
Bran wafer (Featherweight)	1 piece	13
Bravos (Wise)	1 oz.	150
Bugles (Tom's)	1 oz.	150
Cafe (Sunshine)	1 piece	20
Cheese flavored:		
American Heritage (Sunshine):		
Cheddar	1 piece	16
Parmesan	1 piece	18
Better Blue Thins (Nabisco)	1 piece	7
Cheddar sticks (Flavor Tree)	1 oz.	160
Cheese bites (Tom's)	1½ oz.	200
Cheese Doodles (Wise):		
Crunchy	1 oz.	160
Puffed	1 oz.	150
Chee-Tos:		
Crunchy, regular	1 oz.	150
Puffed balls or puffs	1 oz.	160
Cheez Balls (Planters)	1 oz.	160
Cheez Curls (Planters)	1 oz.	160
Cheeze-It (Sunshine)	1 piece	6
Corn Cheese (Tom's) crunchy	1⅝ oz.	280
(Dixie Belle)	1 piece	6
(Eagle)	1 oz.	130
Nacho cheese cracker (Keebler)	1 piece	11
Nips (Nabisco)	1 piece	5
Tid-Bit (Nabisco)	1 piece	4
Chicken in a Biskit (Nabisco)	1 piece	11
Chipsters (Nabisco)	1 piece	2
Club cracker (Keebler)	1 piece	15
Corn chips:		
(Bachman) regular or BBQ	1 oz.	150
Dipsy Doodle (Wise)	1 oz.	160

Food and Description	Measure or Quantity	Calories
(Featherweight) low sodium	1 oz.	170
(Flavor Tree)	1 oz.	150
Fritos:		
Regular	1 oz.	150
Chili cheese flavor	1 oz.	160
Happy Heart (TKI Foods	⅜ oz.	40
Heart Lovers (TKI Foods)	⅜ oz.	40
Korkers (Nabisco)	1 piece	8
(Laura Scudder's)	1 oz.	160
(Tom's) regular	1 oz.	155
Corn Snackers (Weight Watchers)	.5 oz.	60
Creme Wafer Stick (Nabisco)	1 piece	47
Corn Stick (Flavor Tree)	1 oz.	160
Crown Pilot (Nabisco)	1 piece	70
Diggers (Nabisco)	1 piece	4
English Water Biscuit		
(Pepperidge Farm)	1 piece	17
Escort (Nabisco)	1 piece	23
French onion cracker (Nabisco)	1 piece	12
Goldfish (Pepperidge Farm)	1 piece	3
Graham:		
Cinnamon Crisp (Keebler)	1 piece	17
(Dixie Belle) sugar-honey coated	1 piece	15
Flavor Kist (Schulze and Burch)		
sugar-honey coated	1 piece	57
Honey Maid (Nabisco)	1 piece	30
(Rokeach)	8 pieces	120
(Sunshine) cinnamon	1 piece	17
Graham, chocolate or cocoa-covered:		
(Keebler)	1 piece	40
(Nabisco)	1 piece	57
Great Snackers (Weight Watchers)	.5-oz. pkg.	60
Hi Ho (Sunshine)	1 piece	20
Meal Mates (Nabisco)	1 piece	23
Melba Toast (See MELBA TOAST)		
Milk Lunch Biscuit (Keebler)	1 piece	27
Mucho Macho Nacho, Flavor Kist		
(Schulze and Burch)	1 oz.	121
Nachips (Old El Paso)	1 piece	17
Nacho Rings (Tom's)	1 oz.	160
Ocean Crisp (FFV)	1 piece	60
Oat thins (Nabisco)	1 piece	9
Onion rings (Wise)	1 oz.	130
Oyster:		
(Dixie Belle)	1 piece	4
(Keebler) *Zesta*	1 piece	2
(Nabisco) *Dandy* or *Oysterettes*	1 piece	3
(Sunshine)	1 piece	4
Party mix (Flavor Tree)	1 oz.	160

Food and Description	Measure or Quantity	Calories
Peanut butter & cheese (Eagle)	1.8-oz. serving	280
Pizza Crunchies (Planters)	1 oz.	160
Ritz (Nabisco)	1 piece	17
Ritz Bits (Nabisco):		
Regular, cheese or low salt	1 piece	3
Cheese sandwich or peanut butter		
sandwich	1 piece	13
Royal Lunch (Nabisco)	1 piece	60
Rye toast (Keebler)	1 piece	16
RyKrisp:		
Natural	1 triple cracker	20
Seasoned	1 triple cracker	22
Saltine:		
(Dixie Belle) regular or unsalted	1 piece	12
Krispy (Sunshine)	1 piece	12
Premium (Nabisco):		
Regular, low salt, unsalted tops		
or *Premium Plus* whole wheat	1 piece	12
Bits	1 piece	4
Fat free	1 piece	10
(Rokeach)	1 piece	12
Zesta (Keebler)	1 piece	12
Schooners (FFV) whole wheat	½ oz.	70
Sea Toast (Keebler)	1 piece	60
Sesame:		
American Heritage (Sunshine)	1 piece	17
Chip (Flavor Tree)	1 oz.	150
Crunch (Flavor Tree)	1 oz.	150
(Estee)	½ oz.	70
Stick (Flavor Tree):		
Regular	1 oz.	150
With bran or low sodium	1 oz.	160
Toast (Keebler)	1 piece	16
Skittle Chips (Nabisco)	1 piece	14
Snackers (Ralston Purina)	1 piece	17
Snackin Crisp (Durkee) *D&C*	1 oz.	155
Snacks Sticks (Pepperidge Farm):		
Cheese	1 piece	17
Lightly salted, pumpernickel, rye		
& sesame	1 piece	16
Sociables (Nabisco)	1 piece	12
Sour cream-onion stick		
(Flavor Tree)	1 oz.	150
Spirals (Wise)	1 oz.	160
Table Water Cracker (Carr's) small	1 piece	15
Taco chip (Laura Scudder's)	1 oz.	150
Tortilla chips:		
(Bachman) nacho, taco flavor		
or toasted	1 oz.	140

Food and Description	Measure or Quantity	Calories
Doritos:		
Regular	1 oz.	140
Cool Ranch, light	1 oz.	120
Salsa Rio	1 oz.	140
(Eagle) *Del Masa*	1 oz.	150
(Laura Scudder's)	1 oz.	140
(Old El Paso)	1 oz.	150
(Planters)	1 oz.	150
(Tom's)	1½ oz.	210
Tostitos:		
Jalapeño & cheese	1 oz.	150
Traditional	1 oz.	140
Town House Cracker (Keebler)	1 piece	16
Triscuit (Nabisco) regular	1 piece	20
Tuc (Keebler)	1 piece	23
Twigs (Nabisco)	1 piece	14
Uneeda Biscuit (Nabisco) unsalted top	1 piece	30
Unsalted (Featherweight)	2 sections (½ cracker)	30
Waverly (Nabisco)	1 piece	17
Wheat (Pepperidge Farm) cracked or hearty	1 piece	25
Wheatmeal Biscuit (Carr's) small	1 piece	42
Wheat Nuts (Flavor Tree)	1 oz.	200
Wheat Snack (Dixie Belle)	1 piece	9
Wheat Snax (Estee)	1 oz.	100
Wheat Snaz (Estee)	1 oz.	110
Wheatsworth (Nabisco)	1 piece	17
Wheat Thins (Nabisco) nutty	1 piece	11
Wheat Toast (Keebler)	1 piece	15
CRACKER CRUMBS, graham:		
(Nabisco)	2 T.	80
(Sunshine)	½ cup	275
CRACKER MEAL (Nabisco)	2 T.	50
CRANAPPLE JUICE (Ocean Spray) canned:		
Regular	6 fl. oz.	127
Dietetic	6 fl. oz.	41
CRANBERRY, fresh (Ocean Spray)	½ cup	25
CRANBERRY-APPLE JUICE COCKTAIL, frozen (Welch's)	6 fl. oz.	120
CRANBERRY JUICE COCKTAIL:		
Canned (Ocean Spray):		
Regular	6 fl. oz.	103
Dietetic	6 fl. oz.	41
*Frozen (Sunkist)	6 fl. oz.	110
CRANBERRY SAUCE:		
Home recipe, sweetened, unstrained	4 oz.	202

Food and Description	Measure or Quantity	Calories
Canned (Ocean Spray):		
Jellied	2 oz.	87
Whole berry	2 oz.	93
CRAN-FRUIT (Ocean Spray)	2 oz.	100
CRANGRAPE (Ocean Spray)	6 fl. oz.	130
CRANRASPBERRY (Ocean Spray)	6 fl. oz.	110
CRANTASTIC JUICE DRINK, canned (Ocean Spray) regular	6 fl. oz.	110
CREAM:		
Half & half (Land O'Lakes)	1 T.	20
Heavy whipping:		
(Johanna) 36% butterfat	1 T.	52
(Land O'Lakes) gourmet	1 T.	50
Light, table or coffee:		
(Johanna) 18% butterfat	1 T.	30
(Sealtest) 16% butterfat	1 T.	26
Light, whipping, 30% fat (Sealtest)	1 T.	45
Sour:		
(Friendship):		
Regular	1 T.	27
Regular	½ cup	220
Light	1 oz.	35
(Johanna)	1 T.	31
(Land O'Lakes):		
Regular	1 T.	30
Light, plain or with chives	1 T.	20
(Weight Watchers) light	1 T.	17
Sour, imitation (Pet)	1 T.	25
Substitute (See CREAM SUBSTITUTE)		
CREAM PUFFS:		
Home recipe, custard filling	3½″ × 2″ piece	303
Frozen (Rich's) chocolate	1⅓-oz. piece	146
CREAM OF RICE, cereal	1 oz.	100
CREAM SUBSTITUTE:		
Coffee Mate (Carnation)	1 tsp.	11
Coffee Rich (Rich's)	½ oz.	22
Cremora (Borden)	1 tsp.	12
Dairy Light (Alba)	2.8-oz. envelope	10
Mocha Mix (Presto Food Products)	1 T.	20
N-Rich	1 tsp.	10
(Pet)	1 tsp.	10
CREAM OF WHEAT, cereal:		
Regular	1 oz.	100
*Instant	1 oz.	100
*Mix'n Eat:		
Regular	1 packet	100

Food and Description	Measure or Quantity	Calories
Apple & cinnamon	1 packet	130
Maple & brown sugar	1 packet	130
Quick	1 T.	40
CREME DE BANANA LIQUEUR		
(Mr. Boston)	1 fl. oz.	93
CREME DE CACAO:		
(Hiram Walker)	1 fl. oz.	104
(Mr. Boston):		
Brown	1 fl. oz.	102
White	1 fl. oz.	93
CREME DE CASSIS (Mr. Boston)	1 fl. oz.	85
CREME DE MENTHE:		
(Bols)	1 fl. oz.	122
(Mr. Boston):		
Green	1 fl. oz.	109
White	1 fl. oz.	97
CREME DE NOYAUX (Mr. Boston)	1 fl. oz.	99
CREPE, frozen:		
(Mrs. Paul's):		
Crab	5½-oz. pkg.	248
Shrimp	5½-oz. pkg.	252
(Stouffer's):		
Chicken with mushroom sauce	8¼-oz. pkg.	390
Spinach with cheddar cheese sauce	9½-oz. pkg.	415
CRISP RICE CEREAL:		
(Malt-O-Meal) *Crisp 'N Crackling Rice*	1 cup	108
(Ralston Purina)	1 cup	110
CRISPY WHEATS'N RAISINS, cereal (General Mills)	¾ cup	110
CROUTON:		
(Arnold):		
Bavarian or English style	½ oz.	65
French, Italian or Mexican style	½ oz.	66
(Kellogg's) *Croutettes*	⅔ cup	70
(Mrs. Culberson's) cheese & garlic or seasoned	½ oz.	60
(Pepperidge Farm)	½ oz.	70
CUCUMBER:		
Eaten with skin	8-oz. cucumber	32
Pared, whole	7½" × 2"	29
Pared, sliced	3 slices (.9 oz.)	4
CUMIN SEED (French's)	1 tsp.	7
***CUPCAKE MIX** (Flako)	1 cupcake	150
CUP O'NOODLES (Nissin Foods):		
Beef	2½-oz. serving	343
Beef onion	2½-oz. serving	323
Chicken	2½-oz. serving	343

Food and Description	Measure or Quantity	Calories
Chicken, twin pack	1.2-oz. serving	155
Shrimp	2½-oz. serving	336
CURAÇAO LIQUEUR:		
(Bols)	1 fl. oz.	105
(Hiram Walker)	1 fl. oz.	96
CURRANT, DRIED (Del Monte) Zante	½ cup	204
CURRANT JELLY, sweetened (Home Brands)	1 T.	50
CUSTARD:		
Canned (Thank You Brand) egg	½ cup	135
Chilled, *Swiss Miss,* chocolate or egg flavor	4-oz. container	150
*Mix, dietetic (Featherweight)	½ cup	80
C. W. POST, cereal, hearty granola	¼ cup	128

D

Food and Description	Measure or Quantity	Calories
DAIQUIRI COCKTAIL		
(Mr.Boston):		
Regular	3 fl. oz.	99
Strawberry	3 fl. oz.	111
*DAIQUIRI COCKTAIL MIX:		
(Bacardi) frozen:		
Peach	4 fl.oz.	98
Raspberry	4 fl.oz.	97
Strawberry	4 fl.oz.	102
*(Bar-Tender's)	3½ fl. oz.	177
(Holland House):		
Instant	.56 oz.	65
Liquid:		
Regular	1 oz.	36
Strawberry	1 oz.	31
DAIRY CRISP, cereal (Pet)	¼ cup	120
DAIRY QUEEN/BRAZIER:		
Banana split	13.5-oz. serving	540
Brownie Delight, hot fudge	9.4-oz. serving	600
Buster Bar	5¼-oz. piece	460
Chicken sandwich	7.8-oz. sandwich	670
Cone:		
Plain, any flavor, regular	5-oz. cone	240
Dipped, chocolate, regular	5½-oz. cone	340
Dilly Bar	3-oz. piece	210
Double Delight	9-oz. serving	490
DQ Sandwich	2.1-oz. sandwich	140
Fish sandwich:		
Plain	6-oz. sandwich	400
With cheese	6¼-oz. sandwich	440
Float	14-oz. serving	410
Freeze, vanilla	12-oz. serving	500
French fries:		
Regular	2½-oz. serving	200
Large	4-oz. serving	320
Frozen dessert	4-oz. serving	180
Hamburger:		
Plain:		

Food and Description	Measure or Quantity	Calories
Single	5.2-oz. serving	360
Double	7.4-oz. serving	530
Triple	9.6-oz. serving	710
With cheese:		
Single	5.7-oz. serving	410
Double	8.4-oz. serving	650
Triple	10.63-oz. serving	820
Hot dog:		
Regular:		
Plain	3.5-oz. serving	280
With cheese	4-oz. serving	330
With chili	4½-oz. serving	320
Super:		
Plain	6.2-oz. serving	520
With cheese	6.9-oz. serving	580
With chili	7.7-oz. serving	570
Malt, chocolate:		
Large	20¾-oz. serving	1060
Regular	14¾-oz. serving	760
Small	10¼-oz. serving	520
Mr. Misty:		
Plain:		
Large	15½-oz. serving	340
Regular	11.64-oz. serving	250
Small	8¼-oz. serving	190
Kiss	3.14-oz. serving	70
Float	14.5-oz. serving	390
Freeze	14.5-oz. serving	500
Onion rings	3-oz. serving	280
Parfait	10-oz. serving	430
Peanut Butter Parfait	10¾-oz. serving	750
Shake, chocolate:		
Large	20¾-oz. serving	990
Regular	14¾-oz. serving	710
Small	10¼-oz. serving	490
Strawberry shortcake	11-oz. serving	540
Sundae, chocolate:		
Large	8¾-oz. serving	440
Regular	6¼-oz. serving	310
Small	3¾-oz. serving	190
Tomato	½ oz.	4
DATE (Dromedary):		
Chopped	¼ cup	130
Pitted	5 dates	100
DE CHAUNAC WINE		
(Great Western) 12% alcohol	3 fl. oz.	71
DELI'S, frozen (Pepperidge Farm):		
Mexican style	4-oz. piece	280
Reuben in rye pastry	4-oz. piece	360

Food and Description	Measure or Quantity	Calories
Turkey, ham & cheese	4-oz. piece	270
DENNY'S RESTAURANT:		
BLT	1 order	542
Chef salad	1 order	263
Chicken:		
Sandwich, breast	1 sandwich	830
Steak, fried	1 order	606
Club sandwich	1 sandwich	614
Denny Burger	1 burger	537
Eggs, omelet, made with *Egg*		
Beaters	1 serving	225
Patty melt	1 serving	657
Super Bird	1 serving	600
Turkey sandwich, sliced	1 sandwich	445
DILL SEED (French's)	1 tsp.	9
DINERSAURS, cereal (Ralston Purina)	1 cup	110
DINNER, frozen (See individual listings such as BEEF, CHICKEN, TURKEY, etc.)		
DIP:		
Acapulco (Ortega)		
with cheddar cheese	1 oz.	64
Avocado (Nalley's)	1 oz.	114
Bacon & horseradish (Kraft)	1 T.	30
Bacon & onion (Nalley's)	1 oz.	113
Barbecue (Nalley's)	1 oz.	114
Bean (Eagle)	1 oz.	35
Blue cheese:		
(Dean) tangy	1 oz.	61
(Nalley's)	1 oz.	110
Chili (La Victoria)	1 T.	6
Chili bean (Old El Paso)	1 T.	8
Clam (Nalley's)	1 oz.	101
Cucumber & onion (Breakstone)	1 oz.	50
Guacamole (Calavo)	1 oz.	55
Hot bean (Hain)	1 T.	17
Jalapeño:		
Fritos	1 oz.	34
(Wise)	1 T.	12
Onion (Thank You Brand)	1 T.	45
Onion bean (Hain) natural	1 T.	17
Picante sauce (Wise)	1 T.	6
Taco (Hain)	1 T.	44
DIP 'UM SAUCE, canned (French's):		
BBQ	1 T.	22
Hot mustard	1 T.	35
Sweet 'n sour	1 T.	40
DISTILLED LIQUOR, any brand:		
80 proof (40% alcohol)	1 fl. oz.	65

Food and Description	Measure or Quantity	Calories
86 proof (43% alcohol)	1 fl. oz.	70
90 proof (45% alcohol)	1 fl. oz.	74
94 proof (47% alcohol)	1 fl. oz.	77
100 proof (50% alcohol)	1 fl. oz.	83
DOUGHNUT (See also *WINCHELL'S*):		
Regular:		
(Hostess):		
Chocolate coated	1-oz. piece	130
Cinnamon	1-oz. piece	110
Donettes, powdered	1 piece	40
Old fashioned, plain	1.5-oz. piece	180
Powdered	1-oz. piece	110
(Dolly Madison):		
Regular:		
Plain or coconut crunch	1¼-oz. piece	140
Chocolate coated	1¼-oz. piece	150
Dunkin' Stix	1⅜-oz. piece	210
Gems:		
Chocolate coated	.5-oz. piece	65
Powdered sugar	.5-oz. piece	10
Jumbo:		
Plain or cinnamon sugar	1.6-oz. piece	190
Sugar	1.7-oz. piece	210
Old fashioned:		
Chocolate glazed or powdered sugar	2.2-oz. piece	260
Cinnamon chip, glazed or orange crush	2.2-oz. piece	280
White iced	2.2-oz. piece	300
Frozen (Morton):		
Regular:		
Boston creme	2-oz. piece	180
Chocolate iced	1.5-oz. piece	150
Jelly	1.8-oz. piece	180
Donut Holes	⅓ of 7¾-oz. pkg.	160
Morning Light, jelly	2.6-oz. piece	250
DRAMBUIE (Hiram Walker)	1 fl. oz.	110
DRUMSTICK, ice cream, frozen:		
Ice cream, in a cone:		
Topped with peanuts	1 piece	181
Topped with peanuts & cone bisque	1 piece	168
Ice milk, in a cone:		
Topped with peanuts	1 piece	163
Topped with peanuts & cone bisque	1 piece	150
DULCITO, frozen (Hormel) apple	4 oz.	290
DUMPLINGS, canned, dietetic (Dia-Mel)	8-oz. serving	160

E

Food and Description	Measure or Quantity	Calories
ECLAIR:		
Home recipe, with custard filling and chocolate icing	4-oz. piece	271
Frozen (Rich's) chocolate	1 piece	196
EEL, smoked, meat only	4 oz.	374
EGG, CHICKEN:		
Raw:		
White only	1 large egg	17
Yolk only	1 large egg	59
Boiled	1 large egg	81
Fried in butter	1 large egg	99
Omelet, mixed with milk & cooked in fat	1 large egg	107
Poached	1 large egg	78
Scrambled, mixed with milk & cooked in fat	1 large egg	111
EGG DINNER OR ENTREE, frozen (Swanson):		
Omelet, Spanish style	7¾-oz. meal	250
Scrambled, with sausage & potatoes	6¼-oz. meal	410
*EGG FOO YUNG, dinner:		
(Chun King) stir fry	5 oz.	138
(La Choy)	1 patty plus ¼ cup sauce	164
EGG MIX (Durkee):		
Omelet:		
*With bacon	½ pkg.	310
*Puffy	½ pkg.	302
Scrambled:		
Plain	.8-oz. pkg.	124
With bacon	1.3-oz. pkg.	181
EGG NOG, dairy:		
(Borden)	½ cup	160
(Johanna)	½ cup	195
EGG NOG COCKTAIL		
(Mr. Boston) 15% alcohol	3 fl. oz.	177

Food and Description	Measure or Quantity	Calories
EGGPLANT:		
Boiled, drained	4 oz.	22
Frozen:		
(Buitoni) parmigiana	5 oz.	168
(Celentano) rollettes	11-oz. pkg.	320
(Mrs. Paul's):		
Parmesan	5½-oz. serving	270
Sticks, breaded & fried	3½-oz. serving	240
(Weight Watchers) Parmesan	13-oz. pkg.	285
EGG ROLL, frozen:		
(Chun King):		
Chicken	3.6-oz. piece	220
Meat & shrimp	3.6-oz. piece	220
Shrimp	3.6-oz. piece	208
(La Choy):		
Almond chicken, entree	2 egg rolls	450
Beef & broccoli, entree	2 egg rolls	380
Chicken	.5-oz. piece	30
Lobster	3-oz. piece	180
Shrimp	.5-oz. piece	27
EGG ROLL DINNER, frozen		
(Van de Kamp's) Cantonese	10½-oz. serving	560
EGG SUBSTITUTE:		
Egg Magic (Featherweight)	½ envelope	60
*Scramblers (Morningstar Farms)	1 egg substitute	35
Second Nature (Avoset)	3 T.	42
EL POLLO LOCO RESTAURANT:		
Beans	3½-oz. serving	110
Chicken	2 pieces (4.8-oz. edible portion)	310
Coleslaw	2.8-oz. serving	80
Combo meal	16-oz. serving	720
Corn	3.3-oz. serving	110
Dole Whip	4½-oz. serving	90
Potato Salad	4.3-oz. serving	140
Rice	2½-oz. serving	100
Salsa	1.8-oz. serving	10
Tortilla:		
Corn	3.3-oz. serving	210
Flour	3.3-oz. serving	280
ENCHILADA OR ENCHILADA DINNER, frozen:		
Beef:		
(Banquet):		
Dinner	12-oz. meal	500
Entree	2-lb. pkg	1080
(Fred's) *Marquez*	7½-oz. serving	304
(Hormel)	1 enchilada	140
(Old El Paso)	11-oz. dinner	390

Food and Description	Measure or Quantity	Calories
(Patio)	13¼-oz. meal	520
(Stouffer's) & bean, *Lean Cuisine*	9¼-oz. meal	280
(Van de Kamp's):		
Dinner, regular	12-oz. dinner	390
Entree, shredded	5½-oz. serving	180
(Weight Watchers) ranchero	9.1-oz. meal	300
Cheese:		
(Banquet)	12-oz. dinner	550
(Old El Paso) festive	11-oz. dinner	590
(Patio)	12¼-oz. meal	380
(Van de Kamp's)	12-oz. dinner	450
(Weight Watchers) ranchero	8.9-oz. meal	360
Chicken:		
(Old El Paso):		
Dinner, festive	11-oz. dinner	460
Entree, regular	1 piece	220
(Weight Watchers) suiza	9.4-oz. meal	330
ENCHILADA SAUCE:		
Canned:		
(Del Monte) hot or mild	½ cup	45
(El Molino) hot	1 T.	8
(La Victoria)	1 T.	5
(Old El Paso) hot	¼ cup	27
*Mix (Durkee)	½ cup	29
ENCHILADA SEASONING MIX		
(Lawry's)	1.6-oz. pkg.	152
ENDIVE, CURLY OR ESCAROLE, cut	½ cup	7
ESPRESSO COFFEE LIQUEUR	1 fl. oz.	104

F

Food and Description	Measure or Quantity	Calories
FAJITA, frozen:		
(Healthy Choice) beef	7-oz. meal	210
(Weight Watchers) chicken	6¾-oz. meal	230
FAJITA SEASONING MIX (Lawry's)	1.3-oz. pkg.	63
FARINA:		
(Hi-O) dry, regular	1 T.	46
(Malt-O-Meal) dry:		
Regular	1 oz.	96
Quick cooking	1 oz.	100
*(Pillsbury) made with water and salt	⅔ cup	80
FAT, COOKING:		
Crisco:		
Regular	1 T.	110
Butter flavor	1 T.	108
(Rokeach) neutral nyafat	1 T.	99
Spry	1 T.	94
FENNEL SEED (French's)	1 tsp.	8
FETTUCINI: frozen		
(Armour Classics) *Dining Lite*, & broccoli	9-oz. meal	290
(Green Giant) primavera	9½-oz. meal	230
(Healthy Choice):		
Alfredo	8-oz. meal	270
Chicken	8½-oz. meal	240
(Stouffer's)	½ of 10-oz. pkg.	270
FIBER ONE, cereal		
(General Mills)	½ cup	60
FIG:		
Fresh	1½" fig	30
Canned, regular pack (Del Monte) whole, solids & liq.	½ cup	100
Dried (Sun-Maid), Calimyrna	½ cup	250
FIG JUICE (Sunsweet)	6 fl. oz.	120
FIGURINES (Pillsbury) all flavors	1 bar	100
FILBERT:		
Shelled	1 oz.	180
(Fisher) oil dipped, salted	½ cup	360
FISH AND SHELLFISH, fresh,		

Food and Description	Measure or Quantity	Calories
frozen and canned (See specific names: HADDOCK, OYSTER, etc.)		
*FISH BOUILLON (Knorr)	8 fl.oz.	10
FISH CAKE, frozen (Mrs. Paul's):		
Breaded & fried	2-oz. piece	110
Thins, breaded & fried	½ of 10-oz. pkg.	300
FISH & CHIPS, frozen:		
(Gorton's)	1 pkg.	1350
(Swanson):		
Regular	5½-oz. entree	320
Hungry Man	14¾-oz. dinner	770
(Van de Kamp's) batter dipped, french fried	7-oz. pkg.	440
FISH DINNER, frozen:		
(Banquet) platter	8¾-oz. dinner	450
(Gorton's) fillet in herb butter	1 pkg.	190
(Kid Cuisine) nuggets	7-oz. meal	320
(Morton)	9¾-oz. dinner	370
(Mrs. Paul's) parmesan	½ of 10-oz. pkg.	220
(Stouffer's) *Lean Cuisine,* Florentine	9-oz. pkg.	230
(Weight Watchers):		
Au gratin	9¼-oz. meal	200
Oven fried	7.1-oz. meal	300
FISH FILLET, frozen:		
(Frionor) *Bunch O' Crunch,* breaded	1 piece	140
(Gorton's):		
Regular, crunchy	1 piece	160
Light Recipe, tempura batter	1 piece	190
(Mrs. Paul's):		
Batter fried, crunchy	2¼-oz. piece	155
Breaded & fried, light & natural	1 piece	290
(Van de Kamp's):		
Batter dipped, french fried	3-oz. piece	180
Country seasoned	2-oz. piece	200
FISH KABOBS, frozen:		
(Mrs. Paul's) light batter	⅓ pkg.	200
(Van de Kamp's) batter dipped, french fried	4-oz. piece	240
FISH NUGGET, frozen (Frionor) *Bunch O' Crunch,* breaded	1 piece	40
FISH SANDWICH, frozen (Frionor) *Bunch O' Crunch,* microwave	5-oz. sandwich	320
FISH SEASONING (Featherweight)	¼ tsp.	<1
FISH STICKS, frozen:		
(Frionor) *Bunch O' Crunch,* breaded	.7-oz. piece	58
(Gorton's) potato crisp	1 piece	65

Food and Description	Measure or Quantity	Calories
(Mrs. Paul's):		
Batter fried	1 piece	69
Breaded & fried	1 piece	43
(Van de Kamp's) batter dipped, french fried	1-oz. piece	55
FIT'N FROSTY (Alba '77): Chocolate or marshmallow	1 envelope	70
Strawberry	1 envelope	74
Vanilla	1 envelope	69
FLOUNDER:		
Baked	4 oz.	229
Frozen:		
(Frionor) *Norway Gourmet*	4-oz. fillet	60
(Gorton's) *Fishmarket Fresh*	5 oz.	110
(Mrs. Paul's) fillets, breaded & fried, crispy, crunchy	2-oz. piece	140
FLOUNDER DINNER OR ENTREE, frozen (Le Menu)	10½-oz. dinner	340
FLOUR:		
(Aunt Jemima) self-rising	¼ cup	109
Ballard, self-rising	¼ cup	100
Bisquick (Betty Crocker)	¼ cup	120
(Elam's):		
Brown rice, whole grain	¼ cup	146
Buckwheat, pure	¼ cup	92
Pastry	1 oz.	102
Rye, whole grain	¼ cup	89
Soy	1 oz.	98
Gold Medal (Betty Crocker) all-purpose or high protein	¼ cup	100
La Pina	¼ cup	100
Pillsbury's Best:		
All-purpose or rye, medium	¼ cup	100
Sauce & gravy	2 T.	50
Self-rising	¼ cup	95
Presto, self-rising	¼ cup	98
Wondra	¼ cup	100
FOOD STICKS (Pillsbury) chocolate	1 piece	45
*FRANKEN*BERRY,* cereal (General Mills)	1 cup	110
FRANKFURTER:		
(Eckrich):		
Beef, or meat	1.6-oz. frankfurter	150
Beef or meat, jumbo	2-oz. frankfurter	190
Meat	1.2-oz. frankfurter	120
(Empire Kosher):		
Chicken	2-oz. frankfurter	106
Turkey	2-oz. frankfurter	107

Food and Description	Measure or Quantity	Calories
Hebrew National:		
Beef	1.7-oz. frankfurter	149
Natural casing	2-oz. frankfurter	175
(Hormel):		
Beef	1.6-oz. frankfurter	139
Range Brand, Wrangler, smoked	1 frankfurter	160
(Hygrade) beef, *Ball Park*	2-oz. frankfurter	169
(Louis Rich) turkey	1.5-oz. frankfurter	95
(Morrison & Schiff)	1.7-oz. frankfurter	149
(Ohse):		
Regular, beef	1-oz. frankfurter	85
Wiener:		
Regular	1-oz. frankfurter	90
Chicken	1-oz. frankfurter	85
(Oscar Mayer):		
Bacon & cheddar	1.6-oz. frankfurter	139
Beef	1.6-oz. frankfurter	143
Cheese	1.6-oz. frankfurter	144
Little Wiener	2″ frankfurter	28
Wiener	1.6-oz. frankfurter	144
FRANKS-N-BLANKETS, frozen (Durkee)	1 piece	45
FRENCH TOAST, frozen:		
(Aunt Jemima):		
Regular	1 slice	85
Cinnamon swirl	1 slice	97
(Swanson) with sausage, plain	6½-oz. meal	450
FRITTERS, frozen (Mrs. Paul's):		
Apple	2-oz. piece	125
Clam	1.9-oz. piece	131
Corn	2-oz. piece	73
Shrimp	½ of 7¾-oz. pkg.	242
FROOT LOOPS, cereal (Kellogg's)	1 cup	110
FROSTED RICE, cereal (Kellogg's)	1 cup	110
FROSTEE (Borden):		
Chocolate	1 cup	200
Strawberry	1 cup	180
FROSTS (Libby's):		
Dry:		
Banana	.5 oz.	50
Orange, strawberry or pineapple	.5 oz.	60
Liquid:		
Banana	7 fl. oz.	120
Orange or strawberry	8 fl. oz.	120
FROZEN DESSERT, dietetic (See also *TOFUTTI*):		
(Baskin-Robbins):		
Low, Lite 'N Luscious	½ cup (4 fl. oz.)	80–100

Food and Description	Measure or Quantity	Calories
Special Diet	1 scoop (2½ fl. oz.)	90
Eskimo, bar, chocolate covered	2½-fl.-oz. bar	110
Mocha Mix (Presto Food Products):		
Bar, vanilla, chocolate covered	4-fl.-oz. piece	230
Bulk:		
Dutch chocolate, strawberry		
swirl or vanilla	4 fl. oz.	140
Heavenly hash	4 fl. oz.	160
Toasted almond	4 fl. oz.	150
(SugarLo) all flavors	¼ pt.	135
FRUIT BARS (General Mills) *Fruit Corners*	1 bar	90
FRUIT BITS, dried (Sun-Maid)	1 oz.	90
FRUIT COCKTAIL:		
Canned, regular pack, solids & liq.:		
(Hunt's)	4 oz.	90
(Libby's)	½ cup	101
(Stokely-Van Camp)	½ cup	95
Canned, dietetic or low calorie, solids & liq.:		
(Del Monte) Lite	½ cup	58
(Diet Delight):		
Syrup pack	½ cup	50
Water pack	½ cup	40
(Featherweight):		
Juice pack	½ cup	50
Water pack	½ cup	40
(Libby's) water pack	½ cup	50
(S&W) *Nutradiet:*		
Juice pack	½ cup	50
Water pack	½ cup	40
FRUIT COMPOTE (Rokeach)	½ cup	120
FRUIT COUNTRY (Comstock):		
Apple or blueberry	¼ pkg.	160
Cherry	¼ pkg.	180
FRUIT & CREAM BAR (Dole):		
Blueberry, peach or strawberry	1 bar	90
Chocolate-banana	1 bar	175
Chocolate-strawberry	1 bar	160
FRUIT CUP (Del Monte):		
Mixed fruits	5-oz. container	110
Peaches, diced	5-oz. container	116
FRUIT, MIXED:		
Canned (Del Monte) lite, chunky	½ cup	58
Frozen (Birds Eye) quick thaw	5-oz. serving	150
FRUIT & FIBRE CEREAL (Post):		
Dates, raisins, walnuts with oat clusters	⅔ cup	120
Tropical fruit with oat clusters	⅔ cup	125

Food and Description	Measure or Quantity	Calories
FRUIT JUICE, canned (Sun-Maid)	6 fl. oz.	100
FRUIT 'N APPLE JUICE (Tree Top)	6 fl. oz.	90
FRUIT 'N GRAPE JUICE		
(Tree Top):		
Canned	6 fl. oz.	100
*Frozen	6 fl. oz.	110
FRUIT 'N JUICE BAR:		
(Dole):		
Regular:		
Cherry, peach passion fruit or		
pineapple	1 bar	70
Pina colada	1 bar	80
Raspberry or strawberry	1 bar	60
Fresh lites, any flavor	1 bar	25
Sun Tops	1 bar	40
(Weight Watchers)	1 bar	35
FRUIT & NUT MIX (Carnation):		
All fruit	.9-oz. pouch	80
Deluxe trail mix or raisins & nuts	.9-oz. pouch	130
Tropical fruit & nuts	.9-oz. pouch	100
FRUIT PUNCH:		
Canned:		
Capri Sun	6¾ fl. oz.	102
(Hi-C)	6 fl. oz.	96
(Lincoln)	6 fl. oz.	90
(Minute Maid):		
Regular	8.45-fl.-oz. container	128
On the Go	10-fl.-oz. bottle	152
Chilled:		
(Minute Maid)	6 fl.oz.	91
(Sunkist)	8.45 fl. oz.	140
*Frozen, *Five Alive* (Snow Crop)	6 fl. oz.	87
FRUIT ROLL:		
(Flavor Tree)	¾-oz. roll	80
Fruit Roll-Ups, Fruit Corners	.5-oz. roll	50
FRUIT SALAD:		
Canned, regular pack:		
(Dole) tropical	½ cup	70
(Libby's)	½ cup	99
Canned, dietetic or low calorie:		
(Diet Delight)	½ cup	60
(Featherweight):		
Juice pack	½ cup	50
Water pack	½ cup	40
(S&W) *Nutradiet:*		
Juice pack	½ cup	60
Water pack	½ cup	35
FRUIT SLUSH (Wyler's)	4 fl.oz.	157

Food and Description	Measure or Quantity	Calories
FRUIT WRINKLES, (General Mills) Fruit Corners	1 pouch	100
FRUITY YUMMY MUMMY, cereal (General Mills)	1 cup (1 oz.)	110
FUDGSICLE (Popsicle Industries)	2½-fl.-oz. bar	100

G

Food and Description	Measure or Quantity	Calories
GARFIELD AND FRIENDS		
(General Mills):		
Pouch:		
1-2 Punch	.9-oz. pouch	100
Very strawberry	.9-oz. pouch	90
Roll	.5-oz. roll	50
GARLIC:		
Flakes (Gilroy)	1 tsp.	5
Powder (French's) with parsley	1 tsp.	12
Salt (Lawry's)	1 tsp.	4
Spread (Lawry's) concentrate	1 T.	15
GEFILTE FISH, canned:		
(Manischewitz):		
Fishlets	1 piece	8
Gefilte:		
Regular:		
12 or 24-oz. container	1 piece (3 oz.)	53
4-lb. container	1 piece (2.7 oz.)	48
Homestyle, 12 or 24-oz. container	1 piece (3 oz.)	55
Sweet, 12 or 24-oz. container	1 piece (3 oz.)	65
Whitefish & pike:		
Regular, 12 or 24-oz. container	1 piece (3 oz.)	49
Sweet, 4-lb. container	1 piece (2.7 oz.)	58
(Mother's):		
Jellied, old world	4-oz. serving	70
Jellied, white fish & pike	4-oz. serving	60
In liquid broth	4-oz. serving	70
(Rokeach):		
Natural Broth	2-oz. serving	46
Old Vienna:		
Regular	2-oz. serving	52
Jelled	2-oz. serving	54
GELATIN, dry, *Carmel Kosher*	7-gram envelope	30
*GELATIN DESSERT MIX:		
Regular:		
Carmel Kosher, all flavors	½ cup	80
(Jell-O) all flavors	½ cup	81

Food and Description	Measure or Quantity	Calories
Dietetic:		
Carmel Kosher	½ cup	8
(D-Zerta) all flavors	½ cup	6
(Featherweight) artificially sweetened or regular	½ cup	10
*(Royal)	½ cup	12
GELATIN, DRINKING (Knox) orange	1 envelope	39
GERMAN-STYLE DINNER, frozen (Swanson)	11¾-oz. dinner	370
GIN, SLOE:		
(Bols)	1 fl. oz.	85
(DeKuyper)	1 fl. oz.	70
(Mr. Boston)	1 fl. oz.	68
GINGER, powder (French's)	1 tsp.	6
GINGERBREAD:		
Home recipe (USDA)	1.9-oz. piece	174
Mix:		
(Betty Crocker):		
Regular	⅑ of cake	220
No cholesterol recipe	⅑ of mix	210
(Dromedary)	2″ × 2″ square	100
(Pillsbury)	3″ square	190
GOLDEN GRAHAMS, cereal (General Mills)	¾ cup	110
GOOBER GRAPE (Smucker's)	1 T.	90
GOOD HUMOR (See ICE CREAM)		
GOOD N' PUDDIN		
(Popsicle Industries) all flavors	2⅓-fl.-oz. bar	170
GOOSE, roasted, meat & skin	4 oz.	500
GRAHAM CRAKOS, cereal (Kellogg's)	1 cup	110
GRANOLA BAR:		
(Hershey's):		
Chocolate chip	1.2-oz. piece	170
Peanut butter	1.2-oz. piece	180
Nature Valley:		
Regular:		
Cinnamon or oats 'n honey	1 bar	120
Oat bran-honey graham	1 bar	110
Chewy:		
Apple	1 piece	130
Peanut butter	1 piece	140
GRANOLA CEREAL:		
Nature Valley:		
Cinnamon & raisin, fruit & nut or toasted oat	⅓ cup	130
Coconut & honey	⅓ cup	150

Food and Description	Measure or Quantity	Calories
Sun Country:		
With almonds	1 oz.	130
With raisins & dates	1 oz.	130
GRANOLA CLUSTERS,		
Nature Valley:		
Almond	1 piece	140
Caramel & raisin	1 piece	150
GRANOLA & FRUIT BAR,		
Nature Valley	1 bar	150
GRANOLA SNACK:		
Kudos (M&M/Mars):		
Chocolate chip	1¼-oz. piece	180
Peanut butter	1.3-oz. piece	190
Nature Valley	1 piece	140
GRAPE:		
American, ripe (slipskin)	3½″ × 3″ bunch	43
Canned, dietetic (Featherweight)		
light, seedless, water pack	½ cup	60
GRAPEADE: (Minute Maid)		
chilled or *frozen	6 fl.oz.	94
GRAPE APPLE DRINK, canned		
(Mott's)	6 fl.oz.	100
GRAPE DRINK:		
Canned:		
Bama (Borden)	8.45-fl.-oz.	120
(Hi-C)	6 fl. oz.	96
(Johanna Farms) *Ssips*	8.45-fl.-oz.	130
(Lincoln)	6 fl. oz.	90
Chilled (Sunkist)	8.45 fl. oz.	140
*Mix:		
Regular (Funny Face)	6 fl. oz.	66
Dietetic (Sunkist)	8 fl. oz.	6
GRAPEFRUIT:		
Pink & red:		
Seeded type	½ med. grapefruit	46
Seedless type	½ med. grapefruit	49
White:		
Seeded type	½ med. grapefruit	44
Seedless type	½ med. grapefruit	46
Canned, regular pack (Del Monte)		
in syrup	½ cup	74
Canned, dietetic pack, solids & liq.:		
(Del Monte) sections	½ cup	45
(Diet Delight) sections	½ cup	45
(Featherweight) sections,		
juice pack	½ cup	40
(S&W) *Nutradiet*	½ cup	40

Food and Description	Measure or Quantity	Calories
GRAPEFRUIT DRINK, canned		
(Lincoln)	6 fl. oz.	104
GRAPEFRUIT JUICE:		
Fresh, pink, red or white	½ cup	46
Canned, sweetened:		
(Ardmore Farms)	6 fl. oz.	78
(Libby's)	6 fl. oz.	70
(Minute Maid) On the Go	10-fl.-oz. bottle	130
(Mott's)	10-fl.-oz. container	124
(Texsun)	6 fl. oz.	77
Canned, unsweetened:		
(Ocean Spray)	6 fl. oz.	70
(Texsun)	6 fl. oz.	77
(Tree Top)	6 fl. oz.	80
Chilled (Sunkist)	6 fl. oz.	72
*Frozen:		
(Minute Maid)	6 fl.oz.	83
(Sunkist)	6 fl.oz.	56
GRAPEFRUIT JUICE COCKTAIL,		
canned (Ocean Spray) pink	6 fl. oz.	80
GRAPE JAM (Smucker's)	1 T.	53
GRAPE JELLY:		
Sweetened:		
Bama (Borden)	1 T.	45
(Smucker's)	1 T.	53
(Welch's)	1 T.	52
Dietetic:		
(Diet Delight)	1 T.	12
(Estee)	1 T.	6
(Welch's)	1 T.	30
GRAPE JUICE:		
Canned, unsweetened:		
(Ardmore Farms)	6 fl. oz.	99
(Johanna Farms) *Tree Ripe*	8.45-fl.-oz.	164
(Minute Maid)	8.45-fl.-oz. container	150
(Seneca Foods)	6 fl. oz.	118
(Tree Top) sparkling	6 fl. oz.	120
(Welch's) regular or red	6 fl. oz.	120
Chilled (Minute Maid)	6 fl. oz.	100
*Frozen:		
(Minute Maid)	6 fl. oz.	100
(Welch's)	6 fl. oz.	100
*GRAPE JUICE DRINK, frozen		
(Sunkist)	6 fl. oz.	69
GRAPE NUTS, cereal (Post)	¼ cup (1 oz.)	105
GRAVY, canned:		
Au jus (Franco-American)	2-oz. serving	5
Beef (Franco-American)	2-oz. serving	25

Food and Description	Measure or Quantity	Calories
Brown:		
(Estee) dietetic	¼ cup	14
(Franco-American) with onion	2-oz. serving	25
(Howard Johnson's)	½ cup	51
(La Choy)	2 oz.	140
Ready Gravy	¼ cup	44
Chicken (Franco-American):		
Regular	2-oz. serving	50
Giblet	2-oz. serving	26
Chicken & herb	¼ cup	20
Mushroom (Franco-American)	2-oz. serving	25
Pork (Franco-American)	2-oz. serving	40
Turkey:		
(Franco-American)	2-oz. serving	30
(Howard Johnson's) giblet	½ cup	55
GRAVYMASTER	1 tsp.	11
GRAVY MIX:		
Regular:		
Au jus:		
*(Durkee)	½ cup	15
*(French's) *Gravy Makins*	½ cup	20
Brown:		
*(Durkee) regular	½ cup	29
*(French's) *Gravy Makins*	½ cup	40
* (Knorr) classic	2 fl. oz.	25
*(Lawry's)	½ cup	47
*(Pillsbury)	½ cup	30
*(Spatini)	1 oz.	8
Chicken:		
*(Durkee) regular	½ cup	43
*(French's) *Gravy Makins*	½ cup	50
*(Pillsbury)	½ cup	50
Home style:		
*(Durkee)	½ cup	35
*(French's) *Gravy Makins*	½ cup	40
*(Pillsbury)	½ cup	30
Meatloaf (Durkee) *Roasting Bag*	1.5-oz. pkg.	129
Mushroom:		
*(Durkee)	½ cup	30
*(French's) *Gravy Makins*	½ cup	40
Onion:		
*(Durkee)	½ cup	42
*(French's) *Gravy Makins*	½ cup	50
*(McCormick)	.85-oz. pkg.	72
Pork:		
*(Durkee)	½ cup	35
*(French's) *Gravy Makins*	½ cup	40
*Swiss Steak (Durkee)	½ cup	23

Food and Description	Measure or Quantity	Calories
Turkey:		
*(Durkee)	½ cup	47
*(French's) *Gravy Makins*	½ cup	50
*Dietetic (ESTEE):		
Brown	½ cup	28
Chicken	½ cup	40
GRAVY WITH MEAT OR		
TURKEY, frozen:		
(Banquet):		
Cookin' Bag:		
Mushroom gravy & charbroiled		
beef patty	5-oz. pkg.	210
& salisbury steak	5-oz. pkg.	190
& sliced turkey	5-oz. pkg.	100
Family Entree:		
Onion gravy & beef patties	¼ of 32-oz. pkg.	300
& sliced beef	¼ of 32-oz. pkg.	160
(Swanson) sliced beef	8-oz. entree	200
GREAT BEGINNINGS		
(Hormel):		
With chunky beef	5 oz.	136
With chunky chicken	5 oz.	147
With chunky turkey	5 oz.	138
GREENS, MIXED, canned:		
(Allen's)	½ cup	25
(Sunshine) solids & liq.	½ cup	20
GRENADINE (Rose's) no alcohol	1 fl. oz.	65
GUACAMOLE SEASONING MIX		
(Lawry's)	.7-oz. pkg.	60
GUAVA	1 guava	48
GUAVA FRUIT DRINK, canned,		
Mauna L'ai	6 fl. oz.	100
GUAVA NECTAR (Libby's)	6 fl. oz.	70

H

93

Food and Description	Measure or Quantity	Calories
(Ohse):		
Chopped	1 oz.	65
Cooked	1 oz.	30
Smoked, regular	1 oz.	45
(Oscar Mayer):		
Baked	.7-oz. slice	21
Black pepper	.7-oz. slice	22
Boiled	.7-oz. slice	23
Breakfast	1½-oz. slice	48
Chopped	1-oz. slice	52
Cooked, smoked	¾-oz. slice	22
Jubilee, boneless:		
Sliced	8-oz. slice	232
Steak, 95% fat free	2-oz. steak	58
HAM & ASPARAGUS BAKE, frozen (Stouffer's)	9½-oz. meal	510
HAM & CHEESE:		
(Eckrich) loaf	1-oz. serving	60
(Hormel) loaf	1-oz. serving	65
(Ohse) loaf	1 oz.	65
(Oscar Mayer)	1-oz. slice	66
HAM DINNER, frozen:		
(Armour) *Dinner Classics,* steak	10¾-oz. dinner	270
(Banquet) platter	10-oz. meal	400
(Morton)	10-oz. dinner	290
HAM SALAD, canned (Carnation)	¼ of 7½-oz. can	110
HAM SALAD SPREAD (Oscar Mayer)	1 oz.	59
HAMBURGER (See *BURGER KING, DAIRY QUEEN, McDONALD'S, WHITE CASTLE,* etc; see also BEEF, ground)		
HAMBURGER MIX:		
Hamburger Helper (General Mills):		
Beef noodle or hamburger hash	⅕ pkg.	320
Cheeseburger macaroni	⅕ pkg.	370
Chili, with beans	¼ pkg.	350
Hamburger stew	⅕ pkg.	300
Lasagna	⅕ pkg.	340
Sloppy Joe Bake	⅕ pkg.	340
Make a Better Burger (Lipton) mildly seasoned or onion	⅕ pkg.	30
HAMBURGER SEASONING MIX:		
*(Durkee)	1 cup	663
(French's)	1-oz. pkg.	100
HARDEE'S RESTAURANT:		
Apple turnover	3.2-oz. piece	270
Big Cookie	1.7-oz. piece	250

Food and Description	Measure or Quantity	Calories
Big Country Breakfast:		
Bacon	7.65-oz. meal	660
Country ham	8.96-oz. meal	670
Ham	8.85-oz. meal	620
Sausage	9.7-oz. meal	850
Biscuit:		
Bacon	3.3-oz. serving	360
Bacon & egg	4.4-oz. serving	410
Bacon, egg & cheese	4.8-oz. serving	460
Chicken	5.1-oz. serving	430
Country ham:		
Plain	3.8-oz. serving	350
& egg	4.9-oz. serving	400
'n gravy	7.8-oz. serving	440
Ham:		
Plain	3.7-oz. serving	320
With egg	4.9-oz. serving	370
With egg & cheese	5.3-oz. serving	420
Rise 'N Shine:		
Plain	2.9-oz. serving	320
Canadian bacon	5.7-oz. serving	470
Sausage:		
Plain	4.2-oz. serving	440
With egg	5.3-oz. serving	490
Steak:		
Plain	5.2-oz. serving	500
With egg	6.3-oz. serving	550
Cheeseburger:		
Plain	4.3-oz. serving	320
Bacon	7.7-oz. serving	610
Quarter-pound	6.4-oz. serving	500
Chicken fillet sandwich	6.1-oz. sandwich	370
Chicken, grilled, sandwich	6.8-oz. sandwich	310
Chicken Stix:		
6-piece	3½-oz. serving	210
9-piece	5.3-oz. serving	310
Cool Twist:		
Cone:		
Chocolate	4.2-oz. serving	200
Vanilla	4.2-oz. serving	190
Vanilla/chocolate	4.2-oz. serving	190
Sundae:		
Caramel	6-oz. serving	330
Hot fudge	5.9-oz. serving	320
Strawberry	5.9-oz. serving	260
Fisherman's Fillet, sandwich	7.3-oz. sandwich	500
Hamburger:		
Plain	3.9-oz. serving	270
Big Deluxe	7.6-oz. serving	500

Food and Description	Measure or Quantity	Calories
Mushroom 'N Swiss	6.6-oz. serving	490
Hot dog, all beef	4.2-oz. serving	300
Hot ham 'n cheese	4.2-oz. sandwich	330
Margarine/butter blend	.2-oz. serving	35
Pancakes, three:		
Plain	4.8-oz. serving	280
With sausage pattie	6.2-oz. serving	430
With bacon strips	5.3-oz. serving	350
Potato:		
French fries:		
Regular	2½-oz. order	230
Large	4-oz. order	360
Hash Rounds	2.8-oz. serving	230
Roast beef:		
Regular	4-oz. serving	260
Big Roast Beef	4.7-oz. serving	300
Salads:		
Chef	10.4-oz. serving	240
Chicken & pasta	14.6-oz. serving	230
Garden	8.5-oz. serving	210
Side	3.9-oz. serving	20
Shake:		
Chocolate	12 fl. oz.	460
Strawberry	12 fl. oz.	440
Vanilla	12 fl. oz.	400
Syrup	1½-oz. serving	120
Turkey club sandwich	7.3-oz. serving	390
HEADCHEESE (Oscar Mayer)	1-oz. serving	55
HEARTWISE, cereal (Kellogg's)	⅔ cup (1 oz.)	90
HERRING, canned (Vita):		
Cocktail, drained	8-oz. jar	342
In cream sauce	8-oz. jar	397
Tastee Bits, drained	8-oz. jar	361
HERRING, SMOKED, kippered	4-oz. serving	239
HICKORY NUT, shelled	1 oz.	191
HOMINY, canned (Allen's)		
golden, solids & liq.	½ cup	80
HOMINY GRITS:		
Dry:		
(Albers)	1½ oz.	150
(Aunt Jemima)	3 T.	102
(Quaker):		
Regular	3 T.	101
Instant:		
Regular	.8-oz. packet	79
With imitation bacon or ham	1-oz. packet	101
Cooked	1 cup	125
HONEY, strained	1 T.	61

Food and Description	Measure or Quantity	Calories
HONEY BUNCHES OF OATS, cereal (Post):		
With almonds	⅔ cup (1 oz.)	115
Honey roasted	⅔ cup (1 oz.)	111
HONEYCOMB, cereal (Post) regular	1⅓ cups (1 oz.)	110
HONEYDEW	2″ × 7″ wedge	31
HONEY SMACKS, cereal (Kellogg's)	¾ cup (1 oz.)	110
HORSERADISH:		
Raw, pared	1 oz.	25
Prepared (Gold's)	1 tsp.	4
HOT BITES, frozen (Banquet):		
Cheese, mozzarella nuggets	¼ of 10½-oz. pkg.	240
Chicken:		
Regular:		
Breast patty, regular or southern fried	¼ of 10½-oz. pkg.	210
Drum snackers	¼ of 10½-oz. pkg.	220
Nuggets:		
Plain	¼ of 10½-oz. pkg.	210
With cheddar or hot & spicy	¼ of 10½-oz. pkg.	250
Southern fried	¼ of 10½-oz. pkg.	220
Microwave:		
Breast pattie:		
Regular, & bun	4-oz. pkg.	310
Southern fried, & biscuit	4-oz. pkg.	320
Nuggets, hot & spicy, with BBQ sauce	4½-oz. pkg.	360
HOT DOG (See FRANKFURTER)		
HOT WHEELS, cereal (Ralston Purina)	1 cup	110
HULA COOLER DRINK, canned (Hi-C)	6 fl. oz.	97

I

Food and Description	Measure or Quantity	Calories
ICE CREAM (Listed by type, such as sandwich, or *Whammy*, or by flavor—see also FROZEN DESSERT):		
Almond (Good Humor) supreme	4 fl. oz.	350
Almond amaretto (Baskin-Robbins)	4 fl. oz.	280
Bar:		
(Good Humor):		
Chip candy crunch	3-fl.-oz. bar	255
Chocolate Eclair	3-fl.-oz. bar	187
Halo bar	2½-fl.-oz. bar	230
Shark bar	3-fl.-oz. bar	68
Strawberry shortcake	3-fl.-oz. bar	176
Toasted almond	3-fl.-oz. bar	212
Vanilla, chocolate coated	3-fl.-oz. bar	198
(Häagen-Dazs):		
Chocolate with dark chocolate coating	1 bar	360
Fudge	1 bar	210
Vanilla with milk chocolate coating	1 bar	320
Blueberry & cream (Häagen-Dazs)	4 fl. oz.	190
Bon Bon (Carnation) vanilla	1 piece	33
Brittle bar (Häagen-Dazs)	1 bar	370
Butter Almond (Breyer's)	½ cup	170
Butter pecan:		
(Breyer's)	¼ pt.	180
(Häagen-Dazs)	4 fl. oz.	290
(Lady Borden)	½ cup	180
Cappuccino, (Baskin-Robbins) chip	4 fl. oz.	310
Chocolate:		
(Baskin-Robbins):		
Regular	4 fl. oz.	264
Mousse Royale	4 fl. oz.	293
(Borden) old fashioned recipe	½ cup	130
(Breyer's)	½ cup	160
(Good Humor) bulk	4 fl. oz.	130
(Häagen-Dazs) mint	4 fl. oz.	300
(Howard Johnson's)	½ cup	221

Food and Description	Measure or Quantity	Calories
Chocolate fudge (Häagen-Dazs) deep	4 fl. oz.	300
Chocolate peanut butter (Häagen-Dazs)	4 fl. oz.	330
Chocolate raspberry truffle (Baskin-Robbins)	4 fl. oz.	310
Chocolate swirl (Borden)	½ cup	130
Coffee:		
(Breyer's)	½ cup	140
(Häagen-Dazs)	4 fl. oz.	270
Cookies & cream:		
(Breyer's)	½ cup	170
(Sealtest)	½ cup	150
Cookie sandwich (Good Humor)	2.7-fl.-oz. piece	290
Eskimo Pie, vanilla with chocolate coating	3-fl.-oz. bar	180
Eskimo, Thin Mint, with chocolate coating	2-fl.-oz. bar	140
Fat Frog (Good Humor)	3-fl.-oz. pop	154
Fudge cake (Good Humor)	6.3 fl. oz.	214
Fudge royal (Sealtest)	½ cup	140
Grand marnier (Baskin-Robbins)	4 fl. oz.	240
Honey (Häagen-Dazs)	4 fl. oz.	250
Jamocha (Baskin-Robbins)	1 scoop (2½ fl. oz.)	146
Jamocha almond fudge (Baskin-Robbins)	4 fl. oz.	270
Jumbo Jet Star (Good Humor)	4.5 fl. oz.	84
King cone (Good Humor) boysenberry	5 fl.oz.	340
Key lime & cream (Häagen-Dazs)	4 fl. oz.	200
Macadamia nut (Häagen-Dazs)	4 fl. oz.	280
Maple walnut (Häagen-Dazs)	4 fl. oz.	310
Milky pop (Good Humor)	1.5-fl.-oz. piece	46
Mocha double nut (Häagen-Dazs)	4 fl. oz.	290
Orange & cream (Haägen-Dazs)	4 fl. oz.	200
Oreo, Cookies 'n Cream:		
Bulk	3 fl. oz.	140
Sandwich	1 piece	240
Peach (Häagen-Dazs)	4 fl. oz.	212
Pralines 'N Cream (Baskin-Robbins)	1 scoop (2½ fl. oz.)	177
Rocky Road (Baskin-Robbins)	4 fl. oz.	300
Rum raisin (Häagen-Dazs)	4 fl. oz.	250
Sandwich (Good Humor) vanilla	2½-oz. piece	161
Strawberry:		
(Baskin-Robbins) wild, light	4 fl. oz.	90
(Borden)	½ cup	130
(Breyer's)	½ cup	130
(Häagen-Dazs)	4 fl. oz.	250
(Howard Johnson's)	½ cup	187
Strawberry & cream:		
(Borden) old fashioned recipe	½ cup	130

Food and Description	Measure or Quantity	Calories
(Good Humor)	4 fl. oz.	94
Supreme (Good Humor) milk	4 fl. oz.	278
Vanilla:		
(Baskin-Robbins) regular	4 fl. oz.	235
(Borden)	½ cup	130
(Eagle Brand)	½ cup	150
(Häagen-Dazs)	4 fl. oz.	260
(Howard Johnson's)	½ cup	210
(Land O'Lakes)	4 fl. oz.	140
(Sealtest)	½ cup	140
Vanilla caramel (Häagen-Dazs)	4 fl. oz.	310
Vanilla & caramel triple nut (Häagen-Dazs)	4 fl. oz.	310
Vanilla-chocolate cup (Good Humor)	6 fl. oz.	201
Vanilla cup (Good Humor)	3 fl. oz.	98
Vanilla sandwich (Good Humor)	3 fl. oz.	191
Vanilla swiss almond (Häagen-Dazs)	4 fl. oz.	290
Whammy (Good Humor) assorted	1.6-oz. piece	95
ICE CREAM CONE, cone only:		
(Baskin-Robbins):		
Sugar	1 cone	60
Waffle	1 cone	140
(Comet) sugar	1 cone	40
ICE CREAM CUP, cup only		
(Comet) regular	1 cup	20
***ICE CREAM MIX** (Salada) any flavor	1 cup	310
ICE MILK:		
Hardened	¼ pt.	100
Soft-serve	¼ pt.	133
(Borden):		
Chocolate	½ cup	100
Vanilla	½ cup	90
(Land O'Lakes) vanilla	4 fl. oz.	110
(Light 'n Lively) coffee	½ cup	100
(Meadow Gold) vanilla, 4% fat	¼ pt.	95
(Weight Watchers) **GRAND COLLECTION,** premium:		
Chocolate:		
Regular or fudge	½ cup	110
Chip or swirl	½ cup	120
Fudge marble, pecan pralines 'n cream or strawberries 'n cream	½ cup	120
Neapolitan	½ cup	110
Vanilla, regular or swiss	½ cup	100
***ICE TEASERS** (Nestlé)	8 fl. oz.	6

J

Food and Description	Measure or Quantity	Calories
JACK IN THE BOX RESTAURANT:		
Beef fajita pita sandwich	6.2-oz. serving	333
Breadstick, sesame	.6-oz. piece	70
Breakfast Jack	4.4-oz. serving	307
Burger:		
Regular	3.6-oz. serving	267
Cheeseburger:		
Regular	4-oz. serving	315
Bacon	8.1-oz. serving	705
Double	5¼-oz. serving	467
Ultimate	9.9-oz. serving	942
Jumbo Jack:		
Regular	7.8-oz. serving	584
With cheese	8.5-oz. serving	677
Swiss & bacon	6.6-oz. serving	678
Cheesecake	3.5-oz. serving	309
Chicken fajita pita sandwich	6.7-oz. sandwich	292
Chicken fillet sandwich, grilled	7.2-oz. sandwich	408
Chicken strips	1 piece	87
Chicken supreme sandwich	8.1-oz. serving	575
Coffee, black	8 fl. oz.	2
Egg, scrambled, platter	8.8-oz. serving	662
Egg roll	1 piece	135
Fish supreme sandwich	8-oz. sandwich	554
French fries:		
Regular	2.4-oz. order	221
Large	3.8-oz. order	353
Jumbo	4.8-oz. order	442
Jelly, grape	.5-oz. serving	38
Ketchup	1 serving	10
Mayonnaise	1 serving	152
Milk, low fat	8 fl. oz.	122
Milk shake, any flavor	10 oz.	320
Mustard	1 serving	8
Onion rings	3.8-oz. serving	382
Orange juice	6.5-oz. serving	80
Pancake platter	8.1-oz. serving	612

Food and Description	Measure or Quantity	Calories
Salad:		
Chef	13-oz. salad	295
Mexican chicken	15.2-oz. salad	443
Side	3.9-oz. salad	51
Taco	14.8-oz. salad	641
Salad dressing:		
Regular:		
Blue cheese	1.2-oz. serving	131
Buttermilk	1.2-oz. serving	181
1000 Island	1.2-oz. serving	156
Dietetic or low calorie, French	1.2-oz. serving	80
Sauce:		
A-1	1.8-oz. serving	35
BBQ	.9-oz. serving	44
Guacamole	.9-oz. serving	55
Mayo-mustard	.8-oz. serving	124
Mayo-onion	.8-oz. serving	143
Salsa	.9-oz. serving	8
Seafood cocktail	1-oz. serving	32
Sweet & sour	1-oz. serving	40
Sausage crescent	5.5-oz. serving	585
Shrimp	1 piece (.3 oz.)	27
Soft drink:		
Sweetened:		
Coca-Cola Classic	12 fl. oz.	144
Dr. Pepper	12 fl. oz.	144
Root beer, Ramblin'	12 fl. oz.	176
Sprite	12 fl. oz.	144
Diet, Coca-Cola	12 fl. oz.	Tr.
Supreme crescent	5.1-oz. serving	547
Syrup, pancake	1.5-oz. serving	121
Taco:		
Regular	2.9-oz. serving	191
Super	4.8-oz. serving	288
Taquito	1-oz. piece	73
Tea, iced, plain	12 fl. oz.	3
Tortilla chips	1 oz.	139
Turnover, hot apple	4.2-oz. piece	410
JELL-O FRUIT BAR	1 bar	45
JELL-O FRUIT & CREAM BAR	1 bar	72
JELL-O GELATIN POPS	1 pop	35
JELL-O PUDDING POPS:		
Chocolate, chocolate with chocolate chips & vanilla with chocolate chips	1 bar	80
Chocolate covered chocolate & vanilla	1 bar	130
JELLY, sweetened (See also individual flavors)		

Food and Description	Measure or Quantity	Calories
(Crosse & Blackwell) all flavors	1 T.	51
JERUSALEM ARTICHOKE, pared	4 oz.	75
JOHANNISBERG RIESLING WINE		
(Louis M. Martini)	3 fl. oz.	59
JUST RIGHT, cereal (Kellogg's):		
with fiber nuggets	⅔ cup (1 oz.)	100
with fruit & nuts	¾ cup (1 oz.)	140

K

Food and Description	Measure or Quantity	Calories
KABOOM, cereal (General Mills)	1 cup	110
KALE:		
Boiled, leaves only	4 oz.	110
Canned (Allen's) chopped, solids & liq.	½ cup	25
Frozen:		
(Birds Eye) chopped	⅓ pkg.	32
(Frosty Acres)	3.3 oz.	25
(McKenzie) chopped	3⅓ oz.	30
(Southland) chopped	⅕ of 16-oz. pkg.	25
KARO SYRUP (See SYRUP)		
KEFIR (Alta-Dena Dairy):		
Plain	1 cup	180
Flavored	1 cup	190
KENMAI, cereal:		
Plain	¾ cup	110
Almond & raisin	¾ cup	150
KFC (KENTUCKY FRIED CHICKEN):		
Biscuit, buttermilk	2.3-oz. serving	235
Chicken:		
Original recipe:		
Breast:		
Center	4-oz. piece	283
Side	3.2-oz. piece	267
Drumstick	2-oz. piece	146
Thigh	3.7-oz. piece	294
Wing	1.9-oz. piece	178
Extra Tasty Crispy:		
Breast:		
Center	4.8 piece	344
Side	1 piece	379
Drumstick	2.4-oz. piece	205
Thigh	4.2-oz. piece	414
Wing	2.3-oz. piece	254
Lite 'n Crispy:		
Breast:		
Center	1 piece	220

Food and Description	Measure or Quantity	Calories
Side	1 piece	204
Drumstick	1 piece	121
Thigh	1 piece	246
Chicken Littles	1.7-oz. sandwich	169
Chicken nugget	1 piece	46
Chicken sandwich, *Colonel's*	5.9-oz. sandwich	482
Cole slaw	3.2-oz. serving	119
Corn on the cob	5-oz. serving	176
Hot wings	.7-oz. piece	63
Potatoes:		
French fries	2.7-oz. regular order	244
Mashed, & gravy	3½-oz. serving	71
Sauce:		
Barbecue	1-oz. serving	35
Honey	.5-oz. serving	49
Mustard	1-oz. serving	36
Sweet & sour	1-oz. serving	58
KETCHUP (See CATSUP)		
KIDNEY:		
Beef, braised	4 oz.	286
Calf, raw	4 oz.	128
Lamb, raw	4 oz.	119
KIELBASA (see **SAUSAGE,** Polish-style)		
KING VITAMAN, cereal (Quaker)	1¼ cups (1 oz.)	113
KIPPER SNACKS (King David Brand) Norwegian	3¼-oz. can	195
KIWI FRUIT (Calavo)	1 fruit (5 oz., edible portion)	45
KIX, cereal	1½ cups (1 oz.)	110
KNOCKWURST(Hebrew National)	3 oz.	263
KOO KOOS (Dolly Madison)	1.5-oz. piece	190
KOOL-AID (General Foods):		
Canned, *Kool-Aid Koolers:*		
Cherry or mountainberry punch	8.45-fl.-oz. container	142
Grape	8.45-fl.-oz. container	136
Orange	8.45-fl.-oz. container	115
Strawberry	8.45-fl.-oz. container	135
Tropical punch	8.45-fl.-oz. container	132
*Mix:		
Unsweetened, sugar to be added	8 fl. oz.	98
Pre-sweetened:		
Regular, sugar sweetened:		
Grape	8 fl. oz.	80
Orange, surfin' berry punch	8 fl. oz.	79
Purplesaurus rex, rainbow punch or tropical punch	8 fl. oz.	84

Food and Description	Measure or Quantity	Calories
Dietetic, sugar free:		
Berry blue, cherry, grape or tropical punch	8 fl. oz.	3
Rainbow punch	8 fl. oz.	4
Raspberry	8 fl. oz.	2
KRISPIES, cereal (Kellogg's):		
Plain	1 cup	110
Frosted	¾ cup	110
Fruity marshmallow	1¼ cups	140
KUMQUAT, flesh & skin	5 oz.	74

L

Food and Description	Measure or Quantity	Calories
LAMB:		
Leg:		
Roasted, lean & fat	3 oz.	237
Roasted, lean only	3 oz.	158
Loin, one 5-oz. chop (weighed with bone before cooking) will give you:		
Lean & fat	2.8 oz.	280
Lean only	2.3 oz.	122
Rib, one 5-oz. chop (weighed with bone before cooking) will give you:		
Lean & fat	2.9 oz.	334
Lean only	2 oz.	118
Shoulder:		
Roasted, lean & fat	3 oz.	287
Roasted, lean only	3 oz.	174
LASAGNA:		
Dry:		
(Buitoni) precooked	1 sheet	48
(Mueller's)	1 oz.	105
Canned (Hormel) *Short Orders*	7½-oz. can	260
Frozen:		
(Banquet) *Family Entrees,* with meat sauce	¼ of 28-oz. pkg.	270
(Buitoni):		
Regular	9-oz. serving	342
Al forno	8-oz. serving	327
Meat sauce	5-oz. serving	212
(Celentano):		
Regular	½ of 16-oz. pkg.	370
Primavera	11-oz. pkg.	330
(Healthy Choice) with meat sauce	9-oz. meal	260
(Stouffer's):		
Regular, plain	10½-oz. meal	360
Lean Cuisine:		
With meat sauce	10¼-oz. meal	270
Zucchini	11-oz. meal	260

Food and Description	Measure or Quantity	Calories
(Swanson):		
Hungry Man, with meat	18¾-oz. dinner	730
Main Course, with meat	13¼-oz. entree	450
(Weight Watcher's):		
Garden	11-oz. meal	330
Italian cheese	11-oz. meal	380
LATKES, frozen (Empire Kosher):		
Mini	3-oz. serving	190
Triangles	3-oz. serving	140
LEEKS	4 oz.	59
LEMON:		
Whole	2⅛" lemon	22
Peeled	2⅛" lemon	20
LEMONADE:		
Canned:		
(Ardmore Farms)	6 fl. oz.	89
(Hi-C)	8.45-fl. oz. container	109
(Johanna Farms) *Ssips*	8.45-fl.-oz. container	85
Kool-Aid Koolers (General Foods)	8.45 fl.-oz. container	120
Chilled (Minute Maid) regular or pink	6 fl. oz.	81
*Frozen:		
Country Time, regular or pink	6 fl. oz.	62
(Sunkist)	6 fl. oz.	92
*Mix:		
Regular:		
Country Time, regular or pink	6 fl. oz.	62
(4C)	6 fl. oz.	60
(Funny Face)	6 fl. oz.	66
Kool-Aid, sweetened, regular or pink	6 fl. oz.	65
(Wyler's) regular	6 fl. oz.	61
Dietetic:		
Crystal Light	8 fl. oz.	5
Kool-Aid	6 fl. oz.	4
(Sunkist)	8 fl. oz.	8
LEMONADE BAR (Sunkist)	3-fl.-oz. bar	68
LEMON EXTRACT (Virginia Dare)	1 tsp.	21
LEMON JUICE:		
Canned, *ReaLemon*	1 fl. oz.	6
*Frozen (Sunkist) unsweetened	1 fl. oz.	7
*LEMON-LIMEADE DRINK, *Crystal Light*	8 fl. oz.	4
LEMON PEEL, candied	1 oz.	90
LEMON & PEPPER SEASONING (Lawry's)	1 tsp.	6
LENTIL, cooked, drained	½ cup	107

Food and Description	Measure or Quantity	Calories
LETTUCE:		
Bibb or Boston	4" head	23
Cos or Romaine, shredded or broken into pieces	½ cup	4
Grand Rapids, Salad Bowl or Simpson	2 large leaves	9
Iceberg, New York or Great Lakes	¼ of 4¾" head	15
LIME, peeled	2" dia.	15
*LIMEADE, frozen (Minute Maid)	6 fl. oz.	71
LIME JUICE, *ReaLime*	1 T.	2
LINGUINI, frozen:		
(Healthy Choice) with shrimp	9½-oz. meal	230
(Stouffer's) *Lean Cuisine*	9⅝-oz. meal	270
(Weight Watchers) seafood	9-oz. meal	210
LIVER:		
Beef:		
Fried	6½" × 2⅜" × ⅜" slice	195
Cooked (Swift)	3.2-oz. serving	141
Calf, fried	6½" × 2⅛" × ⅜" slice	222
Chicken, simmered	2" × 2" × ⅝" piece	41
LIVERWURST SPREAD (Hormel)	1-oz. serving	70
LOBSTER:		
Cooked, meat only	1 cup	138
Canned, meat only	4-oz. serving	108
Frozen, South African lobster tail		
3 in 8-oz. pkg.	1 piece	87
4 in 8-oz. pkg.	1 piece	65
5 in 8-oz. pkg.	1 piece	51
LOBSTER NEWBURG, home recipe	1 cup	485
LOBSTER PASTE, canned, (USDA)	1-oz. serving	51
LOBSTER SALAD	4-oz. serving	125
LONG ISLAND TEA COCKTAIL		
(Mr. Boston) 12½% alcohol	3 fl. oz.	93
LONG JOHN SILVER'S RESTAURANT:		
Catfish:		
Dinner	13.2-oz. serving	860
Fillet	2½-oz. piece	180
Catsup	.4-oz. packet	15
Chicken plank:		
Dinner:		
3-piece	13-oz. serving	830
4-piece	14.6-oz. serving	940
Single piece	1.6-oz. piece	110
Children's meals:		
Chicken planks	7.1-oz. serving	510
Fish	6½-oz. serving	440
Fish & chicken planks	8.1-oz. serving	550
Chowder, clam, with cod	7-oz. serving	140

Food and Description	Measure or Quantity	Calories
Clam:		
Breaded	2.3-oz. serving	240
Dinner	12.8-oz. serving	980
Cod, entree, broiled	5.4-oz. serving	160
Cole slaw, drained on fork	3.4-oz. serving	140
Corn on the cob, with whirl	6.6-oz. ear	270
Cracker, *Club*	.2-oz. package	35
Fish, battered	2.6-oz. piece	150
Fish & chicken entree	14-oz. serving	870
Fish dinner, 3-piece	16.1-oz. serving	960
Fish dinner, home-style:		
3-piece	13.1-oz. serving	880
4-piece	14.8-oz. serving	1,010
6-piece	18.1-oz. serving	1,260
Fish & fries, entree:		
2-piece	10-oz. serving	660
3-piece	12.6-oz. serving	810
Fish, homestyle	1.6-oz. piece	125
Fish & more	13.4-oz. entree	800
Fish sandwich, homestyle	6.9-oz. serving	510
Fish sandwich platter, homestyle	13.4-oz. serving	870
Flounder, broiled	5.1-oz. piece	180
Gumbo, with cod & shrimp bobs	7-oz. serving	120
Halibut steak, broiled	4.1-oz. serving	140
Hushpuppie	.8-oz. piece	70
Pie:		
Lemon meringue	4.2-oz. slice	260
Pecan	4.4-oz. slice	530
Potato:		
Baked, without topping	7.1-oz. serving	150
Fries	3-oz. serving	220
Rice pilaf	3-oz. serving	150
Roll, dinner, plain	.9-oz. piece	70
Salad:		
Garden	8.7-oz. serving	170
Ocean chef	11.3-oz. serving	250
Seafood, entree	11.9-oz. serving	270
Side	4.3-oz. serving	20
Salad dressing:		
Regular:		
Bleu cheese	1.5-oz packet	120
Ranch	1.5-oz. packet	140
Sea salad	1.6-oz. packet	140
Dietetic, Italian	1.6-oz. packet	18
Salmon, broiled	4.4-oz. piece	180
Sauce:		
Honey mustard	1.2-oz. packet	60
Seafood	1.2-oz. packet	45

Food and Description	Measure or Quantity	Calories
Sweet & sour	1.2-oz. packet	60
Tartar	1-oz. packet	80
Seafood platter	14.1-oz. entree	970
Shrimp, battered	.5-oz. piece	40
Shrimp, breaded	2.2-oz. serving	190
Shrimp dinner, battered:		
6-piece	11.1-oz. serving	740
9-piece	12.6-oz. serving	860
Shrimp feast, breaded:		
13-piece	12.6-oz. serving	880
21-piece	14.8-oz. serving	1070
Shrimp, fish & chicken dinner	13.4-oz. dinner	840
Shrimp & fish dinner	12.3-oz. dinner	770
Shrimp scampi, baked entree	5.7-oz. meal	160
Vegetables, mixed	4-oz. serving	60
Vinegar, malt	.4-oz. packet	2
LOQUAT, fresh, flesh only	2 oz.	27
LUCKY CHARMS, cereal (General Mills)	1 cup (1 oz.)	110
LUNCHEON MEAT (See also individual listings such as BOLOGNA, HAM, etc.):		
Banquet loaf (Eckrich)	¾-oz. slice	50
Bar-B-Que loaf (Oscar Mayer)	1-oz. slice	46
Beef, jellied loaf (Hormel)	1.2-oz. slice	45
Gourmet loaf (Eckrich)	1-oz. slice	35
Ham & cheese (See HAM & CHEESE)		
Honey loaf:		
(Eckrich)	1-oz. slice	40
(Hormel)	1 slice	55
(Oscar Mayer)	1-oz. slice	34
Iowa brand (Hormel)	1 slice	45
Jalapeño loaf (Oscar Mayer)	1-oz. slice	72
Liver cheese (Oscar Mayer)	1.3-oz. slice	114
Liver loaf (Hormel)	1 slice	80
Luncheon loaf (Ohse)	1 oz.	75
Macaroni-cheese loaf (Eckrich)	1-oz. slice	68
Meat loaf	1-oz. serving	57
New England brand sliced sausage:		
(Eckrich)	1-oz. slice	35
(Oscar Mayer) 92% fat free	.8-oz. slice	29
Old fashioned loaf (Oscar Mayer)	1-oz. slice	62
Olive loaf:		
(Eckrich)	1-oz. slice	80
(Hormel)	1-oz. slice	55
(Oscar Mayer)	1-oz. slice	60
Peppered loaf:		
(Eckrich)	1-oz. slice	40

Food and Description	Measure or Quantity	Calories
(Hormel) Light & Lean	1 slice	50
(Oscar Mayer) 93% fat free	1-oz. slice	39
Pickle loaf:		
(Eckrich)	1-oz. slice	80
(Hormel)	1 slice	60
(Ohse)	1 oz.	60
Pickle & pimiento (Oscar Mayer)	1-oz. slice	62
Spiced (Hormel)	1 slice	75

M

Food and Description	Measure or Quantity	Calories
MACADAMIA NUT		
(Royal Hawaiian)	1 oz.	197
MACARONI:		
Dry:		
Spinach (Creamette) ribbons	1 oz.	105
Whole wheat (Pritikin)	1 oz.	110
Cooked:		
8–10 minutes, firm	1 cup	192
14-20 minutes, tender	1 cup	155
Canned (Franco-American) *PizzOs*	7½-oz. can	170
Frozen:		
(Morton) & beef	10-oz. dinner	245
(Swanson) & beef	12-oz. dinner	360
MACARONI & CHEESE:		
Canned:		
(Franco-American) regular or elbow	7⅜-oz. serving	170
(Hormel) *Short Orders*	7½-oz. can	170
Frozen:		
(Banquet):		
Casserole	8-oz. pkg.	350
Dinner	10-oz. dinner	420
(Birds Eye) For One	5¾-oz. pkg.	304
(Celentano) baked	½ of 12-oz. pkg.	290
(Green Giant) One Serving	5½-oz. entree	230
(Stouffer's)	6-oz. serving	250
(Swanson)	12¼-oz. dinner	380
Mix:		
*(Kraft):		
Regular, plain	¼ box	190
Velveeta, shells	¼ box	270
*(Prince)	¾ cup	268
MACARONI & CHEESE LOAF,		
packaged (Ohse)	1 oz.	60
MACARONI & CHEESE PIE,		
frozen (Swanson)	7-oz. pie	210
***MACARONI SALAD MIX** (Betty Crocker) creamy	⅙ of pkg.	200

113

Food and Description	Measure or Quantity	Calories
MACKEREL, Atlantic, broiled with fat	8½″ × 2½″ × ½″ fillet	248
MAGIC SHELL (Smucker's)	1 T.	95
MAI TAI COCKTAIL MIX (Holland House):		
Instant	.56-oz. envelope	64
Liquid	1 oz.	32
MALTED MILK MIX (Carnation):		
Chocolate	3 heaping tsps.	85
Natural	3 heaping tsps.	88
MALT LIQUOR:		
Colt 45	12 fl. oz.	156
Elephant	12 fl. oz.	212
Kingsbury (non-alcoholic)	12 fl. oz.	60
Mickey's	12 fl. oz.	156
Moussy (non-alcoholic)	12 fl. oz.	50
Schlitz	12 fl. oz.	176
MALT-O-MEAL, cereal	1 T.	33
MANDARIN ORANGE (See TANGERINE)		
MANGO, fresh	1 med. mango	88
MANGO NECTAR (Libby's)	6 fl. oz.	60
MANHATTAN COCKTAIL (Mr. Boston) 20% alcohol	3 fl. oz.	123
MANHATTAN COCKTAIL MIX (Holland House) liquid	1 oz.	28
MANICOTTI, frozen:		
(Buitoni):		
Cheese	5.5 oz.	310
Florentine	2 manicotti	284
(Celentano):		
Without sauce	1 manicotti	85
With sauce	1 manicotti	150
(Weight Watchers) cheese, in tomato sauce	9¼-oz. serving	300
*MANWICH (Hunt's):		
Regular	1 serving	320
Extra thick & chunky	1 serving	330
Mexican	1 serving	310
MAPLE SYRUP (See SYRUP, Maple)		
MARGARINE:		
Regular:		
Heart Beat (GFA)	1 T.	25
I Can't Believe It's Not Butter	1 T.	90
(Imperial)	1 T.	100
(Land O' Lakes)	1 T.	35
(Mazola)	1 T.	100
(Parkay) regular, soft or squeeze	1 T.	101

Food and Description	Measure or Quantity	Calories
(Shedd's)	1 T.	70
Imitation or dietetic:		
(Land O' Lakes):		
Soy oil spread	1 T.	75
With sweet cream:		
Stick	1 T.	90
Tub	1 T.	75
(Parkay)	1 T.	55
(Promise):		
Light, soft or stick	1 T.	70
Extra light, soft	1 T.	50
(Weight Watchers):		
Regular, reduced calorie	1 T.	60
Corn oil spread	1 T.	50
Light spread	1 T.	50
Sweet	1 T.	50
Whipped		
(Blue Bonnet; Miracle; Parkay)	1 T.	67
MARGARITA COCKTAIL:		
Canned (Mr. Boston) 12½ % alcohol:		
Regular	3 fl. oz.	105
Strawberry	3 fl. oz.	138
*Frozen (Bacardi)	4 fl. oz.	82
Mix (Holland House):		
Dry:		
Regular	.5-oz. pkg.	57
Strawberry	.6-oz. pkg.	66
Liquid:		
Regular	1 fl. oz.	27
Strawberry	1 fl. oz.	31
MARINADE MIX:		
Chicken (Adolph's)	1-oz. packet	64
Meat:		
(French's)	1-oz. pkg.	80
(Kikkoman)	1-oz. pkg.	64
MARJORAM (French's)	1 tsp.	4
MARMALADE:		
Sweetened:		
(Home Brands)	1 T.	52
(Keiller)	1 T.	60
(Smucker's)	1 T.	54
Dietetic:		
(Estee; Louis Sherry)	1 T.	6
(Featherweight)	1 T.	16
(S&W) *Nutradiet*, red label	1 T.	12
MARSHMALLOW FLUFF	1 heaping tsp.	59
MARSHMALLOW KRISPIES, cereal		
(Kellogg's)	1¼ cups	140

Food and Description	Measure or Quantity	Calories
MARTINI COCKTAIL (Mr. Boston):		
Gin, extra dry, 20% alcohol	3 fl. oz.	99
Vodka, 20% alcohol	3 fl. oz.	102
MASA HARINA (Quaker)	⅓ cup	137
MASA TRIGO (Quaker)	⅓ cup	149
MATZO (Manischewitz):		
Regular:		
Plain	1-oz piece	129
Egg	1 cracker	132
Miniature	1 cracker	9
Tam Tam	1 cracker	15
Dietetic:		
Tam Tam, unsalted	1 cracker	14
Thins	.8 oz. piece	91
MATZO FARFEL		
(Manischewitz)	½ cup	90
MAYONNAISE:		
Real:		
(Bennett's)	1 T.	110
Blue Plate (Luzianne)	1 T.	100
Hellmann's (Best Foods)	1 T.	100
(Kraft)	1 T.	100
(Rokeach)	1 T.	100
Imitation or dietetic:		
Blue Plate (Luzianne)	1 T.	50
(Estee)	1 T.	50
Heart Beat (GFA)	1 T.	40
Hellmann's (Best Foods)	1 T.	50
(Kraft) light	1 T.	45
(Pritikin) *Sweetlite*	1 T.	50
(Weight Watchers)	1 T.	50
MAYPO, cereal:		
30-second	¼ cup	89
Vermont style	¼ cup	121
McDONALD'S:		
Big Mac	1 serving	560
Biscuit:		
With bacon, egg & cheese	1 order	440
With sausage	1 order	440
With sausage & egg	1 order	520
Cheeseburger	1 serving	310
Chicken McNuggets	1 serving	290
Chicken McNuggets Sauce:		
Barbecue	1.1-oz. serving	50
Honey	.5-oz. serving	45
Hot mustard	1.1-oz. serving	70
Cookies:		
Chocolate chip	1 package	330
McDonaldland	1 package	290

116

Food and Description	Measure or Quantity	Calories
Danish:		
Apple or cheese, iced	1 piece	390
Cinnamon raisin	1 piece	440
Egg McMuffin	1 serving	290
Egg, scrambled	1 serving	140
English muffin, with butter	1 muffin	170
Filet-O-Fish	1 sandwich	440
Grapefruit juice	6 fl. oz.	80
Hamburger	1 serving	260
Hot cakes with butter & syrup	1 serving	410
McD.L.T.	1 sandwich	580
McLean Deluxe	7.3-oz. serving	320
Milk, 2% butterfat	8 fl. oz.	120
Orange juice	6 fl. oz.	80
Pie:		
Apple	1 pie	260
Cherry	1 pie	260
Potato:		
Fried	1 small order	220
Hash browns	1 order	130
Quarter Pounder:		
Regular	1 serving	410
With cheese	1 serving	520
Salad:		
Chef's salad	1 serving	230
Garden salad	1 serving	110
Side salad	1 serving	60
Salad bar:		
Bacon bits	1 packet	15
Chow mein noodles	1 packet	45
Croutons	1 packet	50
Salad dressing:		
Blue cheese	1 packet (.5 oz.)	70
French	1 packet (.5 oz.)	58
1000 Island	1 packet (.5 oz.)	78
Lo-cal vinaigrette	1 packet (.5 oz.)	15
Sausage McMuffin:		
Plain	1 sandwich	370
With egg	1 sandwich	440
Sausage, pork	1 serving	180
Shake:		
Chocolate	1 serving	390
Strawberry	1 serving	350
Vanilla	1 serving	380
Soft drinks:		
Sweetened:		
Coca-Cola, classic	12 fl. oz.	144
Orange drink	12 fl. oz.	133
Sprite	12 fl. oz.	144

Food and Description	Measure or Quantity	Calories
Dietetic, *Coke*	12 fl. oz.	1
Sundae:		
Caramel	1 serving	340
Hot fudge	1 serving	310
Strawberry	1 serving	280
Vanilla soft-serve, with cone	1 serving	140
*MEATBALL DINNER OR ENTREE, canned (Hunt's) *Minute Gourmet*	7.6-oz. serving	331
*MEATBALL SEASONING MIX		
(Durkee) Italian style	1 cup	619
MEATBALL STEW:		
Canned *Dinty Moore* (Hormel)	7½-oz. serving	245
Frozen (Stouffer's) *Lean Cuisine*	10-oz. serving	240
MEATBALLS, SWEDISH, frozen:		
(Armour) *Dinner Classics*	11¼-oz. meal	330
(Stouffer's) with noodles	11-oz. pkg.	480
MEAT LOAF DINNER, frozen:		
(Banquet):		
Cookin' Bags	4-oz. meal	200
Dinner	11-oz. dinner	440
(Morton)	10-oz. dinner	310
(Swanson) with tomato sauce	9-oz. entree	310
MEAT LOAF SEASONING MIX:		
*(Bell's)	4½ oz.	300
(Contadina)	3¾-oz. pkg.	360
MEAT, POTTED:		
(Hormel)	1 T.	30
(Libby's)	1-oz. serving	55
MEAT TENDERIZER:		
Regular (Adolph's; McCormick)	1 tsp.	2
Seasoned (McCormick)	1 tsp.	5
MELBA TOAST, salted		
(Old London):		
Garlic, onion or white rounds	1 piece	10
Pumpernickel, rye, wheat or white	1 piece	17
MELON BALL, in syrup, frozen	½ cup	72
MENUDO, canned (Old El Paso)	½ can	476
MERLOT WINE (Louis M. Martini) 12½% alcohol	3 fl. oz.	63
MEXICALI DOGS, frozen (Hormel)	5-oz. serving	400
MEXICAN DINNER, frozen:		
(Morton)	11-oz. dinner	300
(Patio) fiesta	12¼-oz. meal	470
(Swanson)	16-oz. dinner	580
(Van de Kamp's) combination	11½-oz. dinner	420
MILK, CONDENSED, *Eagle Brand*		
(Borden)	1 T.	64
*MILK, DRY, non-fat, instant (Alba; Carnation; Pet; *Sanalac*)	1 cup	80

Food and Description	Measure or Quantity	Calories
MILK, EVAPORATED:		
Regular:		
(Carnation)	1 fl. oz.	42
(Pet)	1 fl. oz.	43
Filled (Pet)	½ cup	150
Lowfat (Carnation)	1 fl. oz.	27
Skimmed, (Carnation; *Pet 99*)	1 fl. oz.	25
MILK, FRESH:		
Buttermilk (Friendship)	8 fl. oz.	120
Chocolate:		
(Borden) *Dutch Brand*	8 fl. oz.	180
(Hershey's) lowfat	8 fl. oz.	190
(Johanna):		
Regular	8 fl. oz.	200
Lowfat	8 fl. oz.	150
(Land O'Lakes) lowfat:		
Regular	8 fl. oz.	150
With *Nutrasweet*	8 fl. oz.	110
(Nestlé) *Quik*	8 fl. oz.	220
Lowfat:		
(Borden):		
1% milkfat	8 fl. oz.	100
2% milkfat, *Hi-Protein Brand*	8 fl. oz.	140
(Johanna):		
Regular:		
1% lowfat	8 fl. oz.	100
2% lowfat	8 fl. oz.	120
Buttermilk	8 fl. oz.	120
(Land O'Lakes):		
1% lowfat	8 fl. oz.	100
2% lowfat	8 fl. oz.	120
Skim:		
(Borden)	8 fl. oz.	90
(Land O'Lakes)	8 fl. oz.	90
Whole:		
(Borden) regular or high calcium	8 fl. oz.	150
(Johanna)	8 fl. oz.	150
(Land O'Lakes)	8 fl. oz.	150
MILK, GOAT, whole	1 cup	163
MILK, HUMAN	1 cup	163
MILK MAKERS (Swiss Miss):		
Chocolate, malted or strawberry	1 envelope or 1 tsp.	18
*Chocolate, malted or strawberry	8 fl. oz.	100
MILNOT, dairy vegetable blend	1 fl. oz.	38
MINERAL WATER (La Croix)	Any quantity	0
MINI-WHEATS, cereal (Kellogg's)		
frosted	1 biscuit	25
MINT LEAVES	½ oz.	4

Food and Description	Measure or Quantity	Calories
MOLASSES:		
Barbados	1 T.	51
Blackstrap	1 T.	40
Dark (Brer Rabbit)	1 T.	33
Light	1 T.	48
Medium	1 T.	44
Unsulphured (Grandma's)	1 T.	70
MORNING FUNNIES, cereal		
(Ralston Purina)	1 cup	110
MORTADELLA SAUSAGE	1 oz.	89
MOST, cereal (Kellogg's)	½ cup (1 oz.)	100
MOUSSE:		
Frozen (Weight Watchers):		
Chocolate	½ of 5-oz. container	170
Praline pecan	½ of 5.4-oz. container	190
Raspberry	½ of 5-oz. container	150
*Mix:		
Regular (Knorr):		
Unflavored	½ cup	80
Chocolate:		
Dark or milk	½ cup	90
White	½ cup	80
Dietetic:		
(Estee) any flavor	½ cup	70
Lite Whip (TKI Foods):		
Chocolate:		
With skim milk	½ cup	70
With whole milk	½ cup	80
Lemon or strawberry:		
With skim milk	½ cup	60
With whole milk	½ cup	70
(Weight Watchers)	½ cup	60
MÜESLIX, cereal (Kellogg's):		
Crispy blend	⅔ cup (1½ oz.)	160
Golden crunch	½ cup (1.2 oz.)	120
MUFFIN:		
Apple (Pepperidge Farm) with spice	1 muffin	170
Blueberry:		
(Morton) rounds	1.5-oz. muffin	110
(Pepperidge Farm)	1.9-oz. muffin	180
Bran (Pepperidge Farm)	1 muffin	180
Carrot walnut (Pepperidge Farm)	1 muffin	170
Chocolate chip (Pepperidge Farm)	1 muffin	170
Corn:		
(Morton)	1.7-oz. muffin	130
(Pepperidge Farm)	1.9-oz. muffin	180
English:		
Millbrook:		

Food and Description	Measure or Quantity	Calories
Regular	2-oz. muffin	130
Whole wheat	2-oz. muffin	120
(Pepperidge Farm):		
Plain	2-oz. muffin	140
Cinnamon, raisin	2-oz. muffin	150
(Pritikin) raisin	2.3-oz. muffin	150
(Thomas'):		
Regular or frozen or sourdough	2-oz. muffin	133
Raisin	2.2-oz. muffin	153
(Wonder)	2-oz. muffin	130
Plain	1.4-oz. muffin	118
Sourdough (Wonder)	2-oz. muffin	130
MUFFIN MIX:		
*Apple cinnamon (Betty Crocker)	1/12 pkg.	120
*Applesauce, *Gold Medal* (General Mills)	1/6 pkg.	160
Blueberry:		
*(Betty Crocker) wild	1 muffin	120
(Duncan Hines) wild	1/12 pkg.	98
*Blueberry streusel (Betty Crocker)	1/12 pkg.	210
*Chocolate chip (Betty Crocker)	1/12 pkg.	150
*Cinnamon streusel (Betty Crocker)	1/10 pkg.	200
Cinnamon swirl (Duncan Hines) bakery style	1/12 pkg.	195
*Corn:		
(Dromedary)	1 muffin	120
Gold Medal (General Mills)	1/6 pkg.	130
Robin Hood (General Mills)	1/6 pkg.	130
Cranberry orange nut (Duncan Hines)	1/12 pkg.	184
*Honey bran, *Robin Hood* (General Mills)	1/6 pkg.	170
Oat bran:		
*(Betty Crocker)	1/8 pkg.	190
(Duncan Hines):		
Blueberry	1/12 pkg.	97
& honey	1/12 pkg.	129
*Oatmeal raisin (Betty Crocker)	1/12 pkg.	140
Pecan nut (Duncan Hines)	1/12 pkg.	211
MULLIGAN STEW, canned, *Dinty Moore, Short Orders* (Hormel)	7½-oz. can	230
MUSCATEL WINE (Gallo)		
14% alcohol	3 fl. oz.	86
MUSHROOM:		
Raw, whole	½ lb.	62
Raw, trimmed, sliced	½ cup	10
Canned (Green Giant) solids & liq., whole or sliced:		
Regular	2-oz. serving	12
B & B	¼-oz. serving	12

Food and Description	Measure or Quantity	Calories
Frozen:		
(Larsen)	3½ oz.	30
(Ore-Ida) breaded	2⅔ oz.	140
MUSHROOM, CHINESE, dried	1 oz.	81
MUSSEL, in shell	1 lb.	153
MUSTARD:		
Powder (French's)	1 tsp.	9
Prepared:		
Brown (French's; Gulden's)	1 tsp.	5
Chinese (Chun King)	1 tsp.	5
Dijon, *Grey Poupon*	1 tsp.	6
Horseradish (Nalley's)	1 tsp.	5
Yellow (Gulden's)	1 tsp.	5
MUSTARD GREENS:		
Canned (Allen's) solids & liq.	½ cup	20
Frozen:		
(Birds Eye)	⅓ pkg.	25
(Frosty Acres)	3.3 oz.	20
(Southland)	⅓ of 16-oz. pkg.	20
MUSTARD SPINACH:		
Raw	1 lb.	100
Boiled, drained, no added salt	4-oz. serving	18

N

Food and Description	Measure or Quantity	Calories
NATHAN'S:		
French fries	Regular order	550
Hamburger	1 sandwich	360
Hot dog & roll	1 order	290
NATURAL CEREAL:		
Familia:		
Regular	½ cup	187
Bran	½ cup	166
No added sugar	½ cup	181
Heartland:		
Plain, coconut or raisin	¼ cup	130
Trail mix	¼ cup	120
Nature Valley (General Mills):		
Cinnamon & raisin	⅓ cup	120
Fruit & nut or toasted oat	⅓ cup	130
NATURE SNACKS (Sun-Maid):		
Carob Crunch	1 oz.	143
Carob Peanut	1¼ oz.	190
Carob Raisin or Yogurt Raisin	1¼ oz.	160
Tahitian Treat or Yogurt Crunch	1 oz.	123
NECTARINE, flesh only	4 oz.	73
NINTENDO CEREAL SYSTEM		
(Ralston Purina)	1 cup	110
NOODLE:		
Cooked, 1½″ strips	1 cup	200
(Pennsylvania Dutch Brand)		
broad	1 oz. before cooking	105
NOODLE, CHOW MEIN:		
(Chun King)	1 oz.	139
(La Choy)	½ cup (1 oz.)	150
NOODLE MIX:		
*(Betty Crocker):		
Fettucini Alfredo	¼ pkg.	220
Stroganoff	¼ pkg.	240
*(Lipton) & sauce:		
Alfredo, carbonara	¼ pkg.	140
Butter	¼ pkg.	152
Cheese	¼ pkg.	141

Food and Description	Measure or Quantity	Calories
Chicken	¼ pkg.	131
Parmesan	¼ pkg.	143
Stroganoff	¼ pkg.	110
*NOODLE, RAMEN, canned (La Choy):		
Beef or oriental	1½ oz.	190
Chicken	1½ oz.	187
NOODLE, RICE (La Choy)	1 oz.	130
NOODLE ROMANOFF, frozen (Stouffer's)	⅓ pkg.	170
NOODLES & BEEF:		
Canned (Hormel) *Short Orders*	7½-oz. can	230
Frozen (Banquet) *Family Entree*	2-lb. pkg.	800
NOODLES & CHICKEN:		
Canned (Hormel) *Dinty Moore, Short Orders*	7½-oz. can	210
Frozen (Banquet)	10-oz. dinner	350
NUT (See specific type: CASHEW, MACADAMIA, etc.)		
NUT, MIXED:		
Dry roasted:		
(Flavor House)	1 oz.	172
(Planters) salted	1 oz.	160
Honey roasted (Fisher)	1 oz.	150
Oil roasted (Planters) with or without peanuts	1 oz.	180
NUT & HONEY CRUNCH, cereal (Kellogg's)	⅔ cup	110
NUTMEG (French's), ground	1 tsp.	11
NUTRIFIC, cereal (Kellogg's)	1 cup	120
NUTRI-GRAIN, cereal (Kellogg's):		
Almond raisin	⅔ cup	140
Raisin bran	1 cup	130
Wheat	⅔ cup	100

O

Food and Description	Measure or Quantity	Calories
OATBAKE, cereal (Kellogg's)	⅓ cup	110
OAT FLAKES, cereal (Post)	⅔ cup	107
OATMEAL:		
Cooked, regular	1 cup	132
Dry:		
Regular:		
(Elam's) Scotch style	1 oz.	108
(H-O) old fashioned	1 T.	14
(3-Minute Brand)	⅓ cup	160
Instant:		
(H-O):		
Regular, boxed	1 T.	15
Apple cinnamon	1.2-oz. packet	130
Raisin & spice or sweet & mellow	1 packet	150
Oatmeal Swirlers (General Mills):		
Apple cinnamon, cinnamon spice or maple brown sugar	1 packet	160
Cherry or strawberry	1 packet	150
Milk chocolate	1 packet	170
(3-Minute Brand):	½-oz. packet	162
Plain	1-oz. packet	160
Apple & cinnamon	1⅜-oz. packet	210
Maple & brown sugar	1.5-oz. packet	220
Total (General Mills):		
Regular	1-oz. packet	110
Cinnamon raisin	1.8-oz. packet	140
Quick:		
(Ralston Purina)	⅓ cup	110
(3-Minute Brand)	⅓ cup	110
Total (General Mills)	1 oz.	90
OATS & FIBER, cereal (H-O) hot:		
Boxed, dry	⅓ cup	100
Packets:		
Plain	1-oz. packet	110
Raisin & bran	1.5-oz. packet	150
OIL, SALAD OR COOKING:		
(Bertoli) olive	1 T.	120

Food and Description	Measure or Quantity	Calories
(Calavo) avocado	1 T.	120
Crisco	1 T.	125
Heart Beat (GFA) canola oil	1 T.	180
Mazola, corn oil	1 T.	125
Mrs. Tucker's; (Goya)	1 T.	130
(Progresso) extra light, extra virgin or imported	1 T.	119
Sunlite: Wesson	1 T.	120
OKRA, frozen:		
(Birds Eye) whole, baby	⅓ pkg.	36
(Frosty Acres):		
Cut	3.3 oz.	25
White	3.3 oz.	30
(Larsen) cut	3.3 oz.	25
(Ore-Ida) breaded	3 oz.	170
(Seabrook Farms) cut	⅓ pkg.	32
(Southland) cut	⅕ of 16-oz. pkg.	30
OLD FASHIONED COCKTAIL		
(Hiram Walker) 62 proof	3 fl. oz.	165
OLIVE:		
Green	4 med. or 3 extra large or 2 giant	19
Ripe (Lindsay) by size:		
Colossal	.4-oz. olive	9
Extra large or large	.2-oz. olive	6
Medium or small	.1-oz. olive	3
Super colossal	.5-oz. olive	11
OMELET, frozen (Swanson)		
TV Brand, Spanish style	7¾-oz. entree	250
ONION:		
Raw	2½" onion	38
Boiled, pearl onion	½ cup	27
Canned (Durkee) *O & C:*		
Boiled	¼ of 16-oz. jar.	32
Creamed	¼ of 15½-oz. can	554
Dehydrated (Gilroy) flakes	1 tsp.	5
Frozen:		
(Birds Eye):		
Creamed	⅓ pkg.	106
Whole, small	⅓ pkg.	44
(Frosty Acres) chopped	1 oz.	8
(Green Giant) in cheese sauce	½ cup	90
(Larsen):		
Diced	1 oz.	8
Whole	3.3 oz.	35
(Mrs. Paul's) french-fried rings	½ of 5-oz. pkg.	167
(Ore-Ida):		

Food and Description	Measure or Quantity	Calories
Chopped	2 oz.	20
Dried-battered, *Onion Ringers*	2 oz.	140
ONION BOUILLON:		
(Herb-Ox)	1 cube	10
MBT	1 packet	16
(Wyler's) instant	1 tsp.	10
ONION, COCKTAIL (Vlasic)	1 oz.	4
ONION, GREEN	1 small onion	4
ONION SALAD SEASONING		
(French's) instant	1 T.	15
ONION SALT (French's)	1 tsp.	6
ONION SOUP (See SOUP, Onion)		
ORANGE, fresh:		
Peeled	½ cup	62
Sections	4 oz.	58
ORANGE-APRICOT JUICE		
COCKTAIL, *Musselman's*	8 fl. oz.	100
ORANGE DRINK:		
Canned:		
Bama (Borden)	8.45-fl.-oz. container	120
Capri Sun	6¾-fl.-oz. can	103
(Hi-C)	6 fl. oz.	95
(Lincoln)	6 fl. oz.	90
Ssips (Johanna Farms)	8.45-fl.-oz. container	130
*Mix:		
Regular (Funny Face)	8 fl. oz.	88
Dietetic:		
Crystal Light	6 fl. oz.	4
(Sunkist)	6 fl. oz.	6
ORANGE EXTRACT, imitation		
(Durkee)	1 tsp.	15
ORANGE FRUIT DRINK, canned		
(Ardmore Farms)	6 fl. oz.	86
ORANGE FRUIT JUICE BLEND,		
canned (Mott's)	9½-fl.-oz. can	139
ORANGE JUICE:		
Canned:		
(Borden) *Sippin' Pak*	8.45-fl.-oz. container	110
(Johanna Farms)	6 fl. oz.	84
(Land O'Lakes)	6 fl. oz.	90
(Libby's) unsweetened	6 fl. oz.	90
(Minute Maid)	8.45-fl.-oz. container	129
(Ocean Spray)	6 fl. oz.	90
(Tree Top)	6 fl. oz.	90
Chilled (Sunkist)	6 fl. oz.	76
*Frozen:		
(Citrus Hill):		
Regular	6 fl. oz.	90

Food and Description	Measure or Quantity	Calories
Lite	6 fl. oz.	60
(Minute Maid):		
Regular	6 fl. oz.	91
Calcium fortified	6 fl. oz.	93
Reduced acid	6 fl. oz.	89
(Sunkist)	6 fl. oz.	84
ORANGE JUICE BAR (Sunkist)	3-fl. oz. bar	72
ORANGE JUICE DRINK, canned, *Squeezit* (General Mills)	6¾-oz. container	110
ORANGE PEEL, CANDIED	1 oz.	93
ORANGE-PINEAPPLE JUICE, canned:		
(Land O'Lakes)	6 fl. oz.	90
(Texsun)	6 fl. oz.	90
ORANGE-PINEAPPLE-BANANA JUICE, canned (Land O'Lakes)	6 fl. oz.	100
ORCHARD BLEND JUICE, canned (Welch's):		
Apple-grape	6 fl. oz.	100
Harvest	6 fl. oz.	90
Vineyard	6 fl. oz.	120
OVALTINE, chocolate	¾ oz.	78
OVEN FRY (General Foods):		
Chicken:		
Extra crispy	4.2-oz. pkg.	461
Homestyle flour	3.2-oz. pkg.	339
Pork, *Shake & Bake,* extra crispy	4.2-oz. pkg.	482
OYSTER:		
Raw:		
Eastern	19–31 small or 13–19 med.	158
Pacific & Western	6–9 small or 4–6 med.	218
Canned (Bumble Bee) shelled, whole, solids & liq.	1 cup	218
Fried	4 oz.	271
OYSTER STEW, home recipe	½ cup	103

P

Food and Description	Measure or Quantity	Calories
PANCAKE, frozen (Pillsbury) microwave:		
Regular or harvest wheat	1 pancake	80
Blueberry	1 pancake	83
*PANCAKE BATTER, frozen (Aunt Jemima):		
Plain	4″ pancake	70
Blueberry or buttermilk	4″ pancake	68
PANCAKE DINNER OR ENTREE, frozen (Swanson):		
& blueberry sauce	7-oz. meal	400
& sausage	6-oz. meal	460
*PANCAKE & WAFFLE MIX:		
Plain:		
(Aunt Jemima) Original	4″ pancake	73
FastShake (Little Crow)	¼ of pkg.	133
Mrs. Butterworth's, butter flavor:		
Regular	4″ pancake	73
Complete	4″ pancake	63
(Pillsbury) *Hungry Jack:*		
Complete, bulk	4″ pancake	63
Extra Lights	4″ pancake	70
Golden Blend, complete	4″ pancake	80
Panshakes	4″ pancake	83
Apple cinnamon, *Bisquick Shake 'N Pour* (General Mills)	4″ pancake	90
Blueberry:		
Bisquick Shake 'N Pour (General Mills)	4″ pancake	93
FastShake (Little Crow)	⅙ of 5-oz. container	84
(Pillsbury) *Hungry Jack*	4″ pancake	107
Buttermilk:		
(Aunt Jemima) regular	4″ pancake	100
(Betty Crocker) complete	4″ pancake	70
Gold Medal (General Mills)	⅛ of mix	100
(Pillsbury) *Hungry Jack,* complete	4″ pancake	63

Food and Description	Measure or Quantity	Calories
Whole wheat (Aunt Jemima)	4″ pancake	83
Dietetic:		
(Estee)	3″ pancake	33
(Featherweight)	4″ pancake	43
PANCAKE & WAFFLE SYRUP		
(See SYRUP, Pancake & Waffle)		
PAPAYA, fresh:		
Cubed	½ cup	36
Juice	4 oz.	78
PAPRIKA (French's)	1 tsp.	7
PARSLEY:		
Fresh, chopped	1 T.	2
Dried (French's)	1 tsp.	4
PASSION FRUIT, giant, whole	1 lb.	53
PASTA DINNER OR ENTREE, frozen:		
(Birds Eye):		
Continental	5-oz. serving	164
Primavera, For One	5-oz. serving	204
(Celentano) & cheese, baked	½ of 12-oz. pkg.	280
(Green Giant):		
Regular:		
Dijon	9½-oz. pkg.	260
Marinara, One Serving	6-oz. pkg.	180
Parmesan, with sweet peas,		
One Serving	5½-oz. pkg.	170
Pasta Accents:		
Creamy cheddar	⅙ of 16-oz. pkg.	100
Garlic	⅙ of 16-oz. pkg.	110
Primavera	⅙ of 16-oz. pkg.	110
(Stouffer's):		
Carbonara	9¾-oz. meal	620
Mexicali	10-oz. meal	490
Primavera	10⅝-oz. meal	270
(Weight Watchers):		
Primavera	8½-oz. pkg.	260
Rigati	11-oz. pkg.	290
PASTA SALAD:		
*Mix (Betty Crocker) *Suddenly Salads,* Italian	⅙ pkg.	160
*Mix *Salad Bar Pasta* (Buitoni):		
Country Buttermilk	⅙ pkg.	250
Italian Creamy	⅙ pkg.	290
Frozen (Birds Eye) classic, Italian style	½ of 10-oz. pkg.	170
***PASTA & SAUCE,** mix (Lipton):		
Cheese supreme	¼ pkg.	139
Mushroom & chicken	¼ pkg.	124
Oriental, with fusilli	¼ pkg.	130
Tomato, herb	¼ pkg.	130

Food and Description	Measure or Quantity	Calories
PASTINAS, egg	1 oz.	109
PASTRAMI, packaged:		
(Carl Buddig) smoked, sliced	1 oz.	40
Hebrew National, first cut	1 oz.	44
PASTRY POCKETS (Pillsbury)	1 pocket	240
PASTRY SHEET, PUFF, frozen		
(Pepperidge Farm)	1 sheet	1150
PASTRY SHELL, frozen (Pet-Ritz)	3″ tart shell	150
PÂTÉ:		
De foie gras	1 T.	69
Liver:		
(Hormel)	1 T.	35
(Sell's)	1 T.	93
PDQ, milk flavoring		
Chocolate	1 T.	66
Strawberry	1 T.	60
PEA, GREEN:		
Boiled	½ cup	58
Canned, regular pack, solids & liq.:		
(Comstock)	½ cup	70
(Del Monte) seasoned or sweet, regular size	½ cup	60
(Green Giant):		
Early with onions, sweet or sweet with onions	¼ of 17-oz. can	60
Sweet, mini	¼ of 17-oz. can	64
(Larsen) *Fresh-Lite*	½ cup	50
Canned, dietetic pack, solids & liq.:		
(Del Monte) no salt added, sweet	½ cup	60
(Diet Delight)	½ cup	50
(Featherweight) sweet	½ cup	70
(Larsen) *Fresh-Lite,* low sodium	½ cup	50
Frozen:		
(Birds Eye):		
Regular	⅓ pkg.	78
In butter sauce	⅓ pkg.	85
In cream sauce	⅓ pkg.	84
(Frosty Acres):		
Regular	3.3 oz.	80
Tiny	3.3 oz.	60
(Green Giant):		
In cream sauce	½ cup	100
Sweet, *Harvest Fresh*	½ cup	80
(Le Sueur) in butter sauce	3.3 oz.	67
PEA & CARROT:		
Canned, regular pack, solids & liq.:		
(Comstock)	½ cup	60
(Del Monte)	½ cup	50

Food and Description	Measure or Quantity	Calories
(Libby's)	½ cup	56
(Veg-All)	½ cup	50
Canned, dietetic pack, solids & liq.:		
(Diet Delight)	½ cup	40
(Larsen) *Fresh-Lite*, low sodium	½ cup	50
(S&W) *Nutradiet*	½ cup	35
Frozen:		
(Birds Eye)	⅓ pkg.	61
(Larsen)	3.3 oz.	60
(McKenzie)	3.3-oz. serving	60
PEA, CROWDER, frozen		
(Southland)	⅕ of 16-oz. pkg.	130
PEA POD:		
Boiled, drained solids	4 oz.	49
Frozen (La Choy)	6-oz. pkg.	70
PEACH:		
Fresh, with thin skin	2″ dia.	38
Fresh slices	½ cup	32
Canned, regular pack, solids & liq.:		
(Hunt's)	4-oz.	80
(Libby's) in heavy syrup:		
Halves	½ cup	105
Sliced	½ cup	102
Canned, dietetic pack, solids & liq.:		
(Del Monte) Lite, Cling	½ cup	50
(Diet Delight) Cling:		
Juice pack	½ cup	50
Water Pack	½ cup	30
(Featherweight);		
Cling or Freestone, juice pack	½ cup	50
Cling, water pack	½ cup	30
(S&W) *Nutradiet,* Cling:		
Juice pack	½ cup	60
Water pack	½ cup	30
Frozen (Birds Eye)	5-oz. pkg.	141
PEACH BUTTER (Smucker's)	1 T.	45
PEACH DRINK, canned (Hi-C)	6 fl. oz.	101
PEACH JUICE, canned (Smucker's)	8 fl. oz.	120
PEACH LIQUEUR (DeKuyper)	1 fl. oz.	82
PEACH NECTAR, canned		
(Ardmore Farms)	6 fl. oz.	90
PEACH PRESERVE OR JAM:		
Sweetened:		
(Bama)	1 T.	45
(Home Brands)	1 T.	50
(Smucker's)	1 T.	54
Dietetic (Dia-Mel)	1 T.	6

Food and Description	Measure or Quantity	Calories
PEANUT:		
In shell (Planters)	1 oz.	160
Roasted:		
(Beer Nuts)	1 oz.	180
(Eagle):		
Fancy Virginia	1 oz.	180
Honey roast	1 oz.	170
Lightly salted	1 oz.	170
(Fisher):		
Dry, salted or unsalted	1 oz.	160
Honey	1 oz.	150
Oil:		
Blanched	1 oz.	160
Party	1 oz.	170
(Guy's) dry	1 oz.	170
(Planters):		
In shell	1 oz.	160
Shelled:		
Dry, salted	1 oz.	160
Honey	1 oz.	170
Oil:		
Regular or tavern	1 oz.	170
Sweet 'n Crunchy	1 oz.	140
(Weight Watchers)	1 pouch	100
PEANUT BUTTER:		
Regular:		
(Algood) any type	1 T.	95
(Holsum)	1 T.	94
(Home Brands)	1 T.	105
Jif	1 T.	93
(Peter Pan)	1 T.	90
(Skippy) creamy or super chunk	1 T.	95
(Smucker's)	1 T.	100
Dietetic or low sodium:		
(Estee) low sodium	1 T.	100
(Home Brands):		
Lightly salted or unsalted	1 T.	105
No sugar added	1 T.	90
(Peter Pan) creamy	1 T.	95
(S&W) *Nutradiet,* low sodium	1 T.	93
(Smucker's) low sodium	1 T.	100
PEANUT BUTTER BAKING CHIPS (Reese's)	3 T. (1 oz.)	153
PEANUT BUTTER & JELLY (Bama)	1 T.	75
PEANUT, SPANISH		
(Fisher):		
Raw	1 oz.	160
Roasted, oil	1 oz.	170

Food and Description	Measure or Quantity	Calories
(Planters):		
Raw	1 oz.	150
Roasted:		
Dry	1 oz.	160
Oil	1 oz.	170
PEAR:		
Fresh	3" × 2½" pear	101
Canned, regular pack, solids & liq.:		
(Del Monte) Bartlett	½ cup	80
(Libby's)	½ cup	102
Canned, dietetic pack, solids & liq.:		
(Featherweight) Bartlett:		
Juice pack	½ cup	60
Water pack	½ cup	40
(Hunt's) halves	4 oz.	90
(Libby's) water pack	½ cup	60
Dried (Sun-Maid)	½ cup	260
PEAR-APPLE JUICE (Tree Top)	6 fl. oz.	90
PEAR-GRAPE JUICE (Tree Top)	6 fl. oz.	100
PEAR NECTAR, canned		
(Ardmore Farms)	6 fl. oz.	96
PEAR-PASSION FRUIT NECTAR,		
canned (Libby's)	6 fl. oz.	100
PEAR, STRAINED (Larsen)	½ cup	65
PEBBLES, cereal (Post)	⅞ cup (1 oz.)	113
PECAN:		
Halves	6-7 pieces	48
Roasted, dry:		
(Fisher) salted	1 oz.	220
(Planters)	1 oz.	190
PECTIN, FRUIT:		
Certo	.6-oz. pkg.	19
Sure-Jell	1¾-oz. pkg.	170
PEPPER:		
Black (French's)	1 tsp.	9
Seasoned (French's)	1 tsp.	8
PEPPER & ONION, frozen		
(Southland)	2-oz. serving	15
PEPPER, BANANA (Vlasic)		
hot rings	1 oz.	4
PEPPER, CHERRY (Vlasic) mild	1 oz.	8
PEPPER, CHILI, canned:		
(Del Monte):		
Green, whole	½ cup	20
Jalapeño or chili, whole	½ cup	30
(Old El Paso) green, chopped		
or whole	1 oz.	7
(Ortega):		
Diced, strips or whole	1 oz.	10

Food and Description	Measure or Quantity	Calories
Jalapeño, diced or whole	1 oz.	9
(Vlasic) Jalapeño	1 oz.	8
PEPPERMINT EXTRACT, imitation		
(Durkee)	1 tsp.	15
PEPPERONCINI (Vlasic)		
Greek, mild	1 oz.	4
PEPPERONI:		
(Eckrich)	1-oz. serving	135
(Hormel) regular or Rosa Grande	1-oz. serving	140
PEPPER STEAK:		
*Canned (La Choy)	¾ cup	210
Frozen:		
(Armour) *Classics Lite,* beef	11¼-oz. dinner	220
(Healthy Choice) beef:		
Dinner	11-oz. dinner	290
Entree	9½-oz. entree	250
(La Choy) Fresh & Lite, with rice		
& vegetables	10-oz. meal	280
(Le Menu)	11½-oz. dinner	360
(Stouffer's)	10½-oz. serving	330
PEPPER, STUFFED:		
Home recipe	2¾″ × 2½″ pepper with 1⅛ cups stuffing	314
Frozen:		
(Celentano)	12½-oz. pkg.	290
(Stouffer's) green	7¾-oz. serving	200
(Weight Watchers) with veal stuffing	11¾-oz. meal	270
PEPPER, SWEET:		
Raw:		
Green:		
Whole	1 lb.	82
Without stem & seeds	1 med. pepper (2.6 oz.)	13
Red:		
Whole	1 lb.	112
Without stem & seeds	1 med. pepper (2.2 oz.)	19
Boiled, green, without salt, drained	1 med. pepper (2.6 oz.)	13
Frozen:		
(Frosty Acres) diced:		
Green	1 oz.	6
Red & green	1 oz.	7
(Larsen) green	1 oz.	6
(McKenzie)	1-oz. serving	6
(Southland) diced	2-oz. serving	10
PERCH, OCEAN:		
Atlantic, raw:		
Whole	1 lb.	124

Food and Description	Measure or Quantity	Calories
Meat only	4 oz.	108
Pacific, raw, whole	1 lb.	116
Frozen:		
(Banquet)	8¾-oz. dinner	434
(Frionor) *Norway Gourmet*	4 oz. fillet	120
(Mrs. Paul's) fillet, breaded & fried	2-oz. piece	145
(Van de Kamp's) batter dipped, french fried	2-oz. piece	135
PERNOD (Julius Wile)	1 fl. oz.	79
PERSIMMON:		
Japanese or Kaki, fresh:		
With seeds	4.4-oz. piece	79
Seedless	4.4-oz. piece	81
Native, fresh, flesh only	4-oz. serving	144
PETITE SIRAH WINE (Louis M. Martini) 12% alcohol	3 fl. oz.	61
PHEASANT, raw, meat only	4-oz. serving	184
PICKLE:		
Cucumber, fresh or bread & butter:		
(Fannings)	1.2-oz. serving	17
(Featherweight) low sodium	1-oz. pickle	12
(Vlasic):		
Chips	1 oz.	7
Stix, sweet butter	1 oz.	5
Dill:		
(Featherweight) low sodium, whole	1-oz. serving	4
(Smucker's):		
Hamburger, sliced	1 slice	Tr.
Polish, whole	3½″ pickle	8
(Vlasic):		
Original	1 oz.	2
No garlic	1 oz.	4
Hamburger (Vlasic) chips	1-oz. serving	2
Hot & spicy (Vlasic) garden mix	1 oz.	4
Kosher dill:		
(Claussen) halves or whole	2-oz. serving	7
(Featherweight) low sodium	1-oz. serving	4
(Smucker's):		
Baby	2¾″-long pickle	4
Whole	3½″-long pickle	8
(Vlasic)	1 oz.	4
Sweet:		
(Nalley's) *Nubbins*	1-oz. serving	28
(Smucker's):		
Gherkins	2″-long pickle	15
Whole	2½″-long pickle	18

Food and Description	Measure or Quantity	Calories
(Vlasic)	1 oz.	30
Sweet & sour (Claussen) slices	1 slice	3
PIE:		
Regular, non-frozen:		
Apple:		
Home recipe, two crust	⅙ of 9″ pie	404
(Dolly Madison)	4½-oz. pie	490
Banana, home recipe, cream or custard	⅙ of 9″ pie	336
Blackberry, home recipe, two-crust	⅙ of 9″ pie	384
Blueberry:		
Home recipe, two-crust	⅙ of 9″ pie	382
(Dolly Madison)	4½-oz. pie	430
Boston cream, home recipe	1/12 of 8″ pie	208
Butterscotch, home recipe, one-crust	⅙ of 9″ pie	406
Cherry:		
Home recipe, two-crust	⅙ of 9″ pie	412
(Dolly Madison) regular	4½-oz. pie	470
Chocolate (Dolly Madison):		
Regular	4½-oz. pie	560
Pudding	4½-oz. pie	500
Chocolate chiffon, home recipe	⅙ of 9″ pie	459
Chocolate meringue, home recipe	⅙ of 9″ pie	353
Coconut custard, home recipe	⅙ of 9″ pie	357
Lemon meringue, home recipe, one-crust	⅙ of 9″ pie	357
Mince, home recipe, two-crust	⅙ of 9″ pie	428
Peach (Dolly Madison)	4½-oz. pie	460
Pumpkin, home recipe, one-crust	⅙ of 9″ pie	321
Raisin, home recipe, two-crust	⅙ of 9″ pie	427
Vanilla (Dolly Madison) pudding	4½-oz. pie	500
Frozen:		
Apple:		
(Banquet) family size	⅙ of 20-oz. pie	250
(Mrs. Smith's):		
Regular:		
Plain	⅛ of 8″ pie	220
Dutch	⅛ of 10″ pie	430
Natural Juice, dutch	⅛ of 9″ pie	380
Pie in Minutes	⅛ of 25-oz. pie	210
(Pet-Ritz))	⅙ of 26-oz. pie	330
(Weight Watchers)	3½ oz.	200
Banana cream:		
(Banquet)	⅙ of 14-oz. pie	180
(Pet-Ritz)	⅙ of 14-oz. pie	170
Blackberry (Banquet)	⅙ of 20-oz. pie	270

Food and Description	Measure or Quantity	Calories
Blueberry:		
(Banquet)	⅙ of 20-oz. pie	266
(Mrs. Smith's):		
Regular	⅛ of 26-oz. pie	210
Pie in Minutes	⅛ of 25-oz. pie	220
(Pet-Ritz)	⅙ of 26-oz. pie	370
Cherry:		
(Banquet)	⅙ of 20-oz. pie	250
(Mrs. Smith's):		
Regular	⅛ of 46-oz. pie	390
Natural Juice	⅛ of 36.8-oz pie	350
(Pet-Ritz)	⅙ of 26-oz. pie	300
Chocolate cream:		
(Banquet)	⅙ of 14-oz. pie	190
(Pet-Ritz)	⅙ of 14-oz. pie	190
Coconut cream (Banquet)	⅙ of 14-oz. pie	190
Coconut custard (Mrs. Smith's):	⅛ of 25-oz. pie	180
Custard, egg (Pet-Ritz)	⅙ of 24-oz. pie	200
Lemon cream:		
(Banquet)	⅙ of 14-oz. pie	168
(Pet-Ritz)	⅙ of 14-oz. pie	190
Mince:		
(Banquet)	⅙ of 20-oz. pie	260
(Mrs. Smith's)	⅛ of 46-oz. pie	430
(Pet-Ritz)	⅙ of 26-oz. pie	280
Peach:		
(Banquet)	⅙ of 20-oz. pie	245
(Mrs. Smith's):		
Regular	⅛ of 46-oz. pie	360
Natural Juice	⅛ of 36.8-oz. pie	330
(Pet-Ritz)	⅙ of 26-oz. pie	320
Pumpkin:		
(Banquet)	⅙ of 20-oz. pie	200
(Mrs. Smith's) *Pie In Minutes*	⅛ of 25-oz. pie	190
Strawberry cream (Banquet)	⅙ of 14-oz. pie	170
PIECRUST:		
Home recipe, 9″ pie	1 crust	900
Frozen:		
(Empire Kosher)	7-oz. shell	1001
(Mrs. Smith's):		
8″ shell	10 oz.	640
9″ shell, shallow	10 oz.	640
9⅝″ shell	15 oz.	960
(Oronoque):		
Regular	7.4 oz.	1020
Deep dish	8½ oz.	1200
(Pet-Ritz):		
Regular	⅙ of 5-oz. pkg.	110

Food and Description	Measure or Quantity	Calories
Deep dish:		
Regular	⅙ of 6-oz. pkg.	130
All vegetable shortening	⅙ of 6-oz. pkg.	140
Graham cracker	⅙ of 5-oz. pkg.	110
Refrigerated (Pillsbury)	2 crusts	1920
*PIECRUST MIX:		
(Betty Crocker):		
Regular	1/16 pkg.	120
Stick	⅛ stick	120
(Flako)	⅙ of 9″ pie shell	245
(Pillsbury) mix or stick	⅙ of 2-crust pie	270
PIE FILLING (See also PUDDING OR PIE FILLING):		
Apple:		
(Comstock)	⅙ of 21-oz. can	110
(Thank You Brand)	3½ oz.	91
(White House)	½ cup	163
Apple rings or slices (See APPLE, canned)		
Apricot (Comstock)	⅙ of 21-oz. can	110
Banana cream (Comstock)	⅙ of 21-oz. can	110
Blueberry (Comstock)	⅙ of 21-oz. can	120
Cherry (White House)	3½ oz.	99
Coconut cream (Comstock)	⅙ of 21-oz. can	120
Coconut custard, home recipe, made with egg yolk & milk	5 oz. (inc. crust)	288
Lemon (Comstock)	⅙ of 21-oz. can	160
Mincemeat (Comstock)	½ of 21-oz. can	170
Peach (White House)	½ cup	158
Pumpkin (Libby's) (See also PUMPKIN, canned)	1 cup	210
Raisin (Comstock)	⅙ of 21-oz. can	140
*PIE MIX:		
Boston Cream (Betty Crocker)	⅛ of pie	270
Chocolate (Royal)	⅛ of pie	260
PIEROGIES, frozen:		
(Empire Kosher):		
Cheese	1½ oz.	110
Onion	1½ oz.	90
(Mrs. Paul's) potato & cheese	1 piece	90
PIGS FEET, pickled	4-oz. serving	226
PIMIENTO, canned:		
(Dromedary) drained	1-oz. serving	10
(Ortega)	¼ cup	6
(Sunshine) diced or sliced	1 T.	4
PIÑA COLADA (Mr. Boston) 12½% alcohol	3 fl. oz.	249
PIÑA COLADA MIX:		
*(Bacardi) frozen	4 fl. oz.	110

Food and Description	Measure or Quantity	Calories
*(Bar-Tender's) (Holland House):	5 fl. oz.	254
Dry mix	.56-oz. pkg.	82
Liquid mix	1 fl. oz.	33
PINEAPPLE:		
Fresh, chunks	½ cup	52
Canned, regular pack, solids & liq.:		
(Del Monte) slices, syrup pack	½ cup	90
(Dole):		
Juice pack, chunk, crushed or sliced	½ cup	70
Heavy syrup, chunk, crushed or sliced	½ cup	90
Canned, unsweetened or dietetic, solids & liq.:		
(Diet Delight) juice pack	½ cup	70
(Libby's) Lite	½ cup	60
(S&W) *Nutradiet*	1 slice	30
PINEAPPLE & GRAPEFRUIT JUICE DRINK, canned:		
(Del Monte) regular or pink	6 fl. oz.	90
(Dole) pink	6 fl. oz.	101
(Texsun)	6 fl. oz.	91
PINEAPPLE, CANDIED	1-oz. serving	90
PINEAPPLE FLAVORING, imitation (Durkee)	1 tsp.	6
***PINEAPPLE GRAPEFRUIT JUICE,** frozen (Dole)	6 fl. oz.	90
PINEAPPLE JUICE:		
Canned:		
(Ardmore Farms)	6 fl. oz.	102
(Dole)	6 fl. oz.	100
(Minute Maid) On the Go	10-fl.-oz. bottle	165
(Mott's)	9.5-fl.-oz. can	169
(Tree Top)	6 fl. oz.	100
*Frozen (Minute Maid)	6 fl. oz.	99
PINEAPPLE-ORANGE JUICE:		
Canned:		
(Dole)	6 fl. oz.	100
(Johanna Farms) *Tree Ripe*	8.45-fl.-oz. container	132
*Frozen (Minute Maid)	6 fl. oz.	98
PINEAPPLE PRESERVE OR JAM, sweetened (Home Brands)	1 T.	52
PINE NUT, pignolias, shelled	1 oz.	156
PINOT CHARDONNAY WINE (Paul Masson) 12% alcohol	3 fl. oz.	71
PISTACHIO NUT:		
In shell	½ cup	197

Food and Description	Measure or Quantity	Calories
Shelled	¼ cup	184
(Fisher) shelled, roasted, salted	1 oz.	174
PIZZA PIE (See also *SHAKEY'S*):		
Regular, non-frozen:		
Home recipe	⅛ of 14" pie	177
(*Domino's*):		
Beef, ground:		
Plain:		
12" pizza (small)	1 slice	216
16" pizza (large)	1 slice	303
With pepperoni:		
12" pizza (small)	1 slice	216
16" pizza (large)	1 slice	303
Cheese:		
Plain:		
12" pizza (small)	1 slice	157
16" pizza (large)	1 slice	239
Double cheese:		
12" pizza (small)	1 slice	240
16" pizza (large)	1 slice	350
Double, with pepperoni		
12" pizza (small)	1 slice	227
16" pizza (large)	1 slice	389
Mushroom & sausage:		
12" pizza (small)	1 slice	183
16" pizza (large)	1 slice	266
Pepperoni:		
Plain:		
12" pizza (small)	1 slice	192
16" pizza (large)	1 slice	278
With mushrooms:		
12" pizza (small)	1 slice	194
16" pizza (large)	1 slice	280
With sausage:		
12" pizza (small)	1 slice	215
16" pizza (large)	1 slice	303
Sausage:		
12" pizza (small)	1 slice	180
16" pizza (large)	1 slice	264
(*Godfather's*):		
Cheese:		
Original:		
Mini	¼ of pizza (2.8 oz.)	190
Small	⅙ of pizza (3.6 oz.)	240
Medium	⅛ of pizza (4½ oz.)	270
Large:		
Regular	1/10 of pizza (4.4 oz.)	297
Hot slice	⅛ of pizza (5½ oz.)	370

Food and Description	Measure or Quantity	Calories
Stuffed:		
Small	⅙ of pizza (4.4 oz.)	310
Medium	⅛ of pizza (4.8 oz.)	350
Large	¹⁄₁₀ of pizza (5.2 oz.)	381
Thin crust:		
Small	⅙ of pizza (2.6 oz.)	180
Medium	⅛ of pizza (3 oz.)	210
Large	¹⁄₁₀ of pizza (3.4 oz.)	228
Combo:		
Original:		
Mini	¼ of pizza (3.8 oz.)	240
Small	⅙ of pizza (5.6 oz.)	360
Medium	⅛ of pizza (6.2 oz.)	400
Large:		
Regular	¹⁄₁₀ of pizza (6.8 oz.)	437
Hot slice	⅛ of pizza (8.5 oz.)	550
Stuffed:		
Small	⅙ of pizza (6.3 oz.)	430
Medium	⅛ of pizza (7 oz.)	480
Large	¹⁄₁₀ of pizza (7.6 oz.)	521
Thin crust:		
Small	⅙ of pizza (4.3 oz.)	270
Medium	⅛ of pizza (4.9 oz.)	310
Large	¹⁄₁₀ of pizza (5.4 oz.)	336
Frozen:		
Bacon (Totino's)	½ of 10-oz. pie	370
Bagel (Empire Kosher)	2-oz. serving	140
Canadian style bacon:		
(Jeno's) crisp 'n tasty	½ of 7.7-oz. pie	250
(Stouffer's) french bread	½ of 11⅝-oz. pkg.	360
(Totino's)	½ of 10.2-oz. pkg.	310
Cheese:		
(Celentano):		
Mini slice	1 slice	150
Thick crust	⅓ of 13-oz. pie	290
(Empire Kosher):		
Regular	⅓ of 10-oz. pie	195
3-pack	⅑ of 27-oz. pie	215
(Jeno's) 4-pack	¼ of 8.9-oz. pkg.	160
(Kid Cuisine)	6½-oz. pkg.	240
(Pappalo's) french bread	5.7-oz. piece	360
(Pillsbury) microwave, regular	½ of 7.1-oz. pie	240
(Stouffer's) french bread:		
Regular, double cheese	½ of 11¾-oz. pkg.	410
Lean Cuisine, extra cheese	5½-oz. serving	350
(Weight Watchers) regular	5¾-oz. pie	310
Combination:		
(Jeno's) crisp 'n tasty	½ of 7.8-oz. pie	300
(Pappalo's) pan	⅙ of 26½-oz. pie	340

Food and Description	Measure or Quantity	Calories
(Pillsbury) microwave	½ of 9-oz. pie	310
(Totino's) *My Classic*, deluxe	⅙ of 22½-oz. pie	270
(Weight Watchers) deluxe	6¾-oz. pkg.	300
Deluxe:		
(Banquet) *Zap*, french bread	4.8-oz. serving	330
(Stouffer's) *Lean Cuisine*	6½-oz. serving	350
(Weight Watchers) french bread	6.1-oz. pkg.	310
English muffin (Empire Kosher)	2-oz. serving	140
Hamburger:		
(Fox Deluxe)	½ of 7.6-oz. pie	260
(Jeno's) 4-pack	¼ of 10-oz. pkg.	180
(Pappalo's) thin crust	⅙ of 22-oz. pie	240
(Stouffer's) french bread	½ of 12¼-oz. pkg.	410
Pepperoni:		
(Banquet) *Zap*, french bread	4½-oz. serving	350
(Fox Deluxe)	½ of 7-oz. pie	250
(Jeno's) 4-pack	¼ of 9.2-oz. pkg.	170
(Pillsbury) microwave, regular	½ of 8½-oz. pie	300
(Totino's):		
Microwave, small	4-oz. pie	280
Party	½ of 10.2-oz. pie	370
(Weight Watchers) french bread	5¼-oz. pkg.	310
Sausage:		
(Fox Deluxe)	½ of 7.2-oz. pie	260
(Jeno's) crisp 'n tasty	½ of 7.8-oz. pie	300
(Pappalo's) pan	⅙ of 26.3-oz. pie	360
(Pillsbury) microwave, regular	½ of 8¾-oz. pie	280
(Stouffer's) french bread	½ of 12-oz. pkg.	420
(Weight Watchers)	6¼-oz. pkg.	310
Sausage & mushroom:		
(Celeste)	¼ of 24-oz. pie	365
(Stouffer's) french bread	½ of 12½-oz. pkg.	410
Sausage & pepperoni (Stouffer's) french bread	½ of 12½-oz. pkg.	450
Sicilian style (Celeste) deluxe	¼ of 26-oz. pie	408
Supreme (Celeste) without meat	½ of 8-oz. pie	217
Vegetable (Stouffer's) french bread	½ of 12¾-oz. pkg.	420
*Mix (Ragú) *Pizza Quick*	¼ of pie	300
PIZZA PIE CRUST:		
*Mix, *Gold Medal* (General Mills)	⅙ pkg.	110
Refrigerated (Pillsbury)	⅛ of crust	90
PIZZA ROLL, frozen (Jeno's):		
Cheese	½ of 6-oz. pkg.	240
Hamburger	½ of 6-oz. pkg.	240
Sausage & pepperoni:		
Regular	½ of 6-oz. pkg.	230
Microwave	⅓ of 9-oz. pkg.	250
PIZZA SAUCE:		
(Contadina):		
Regular or with cheese	½ cup	80

Food and Description	Measure or Quantity	Calories
With pepperoni	½ cup	90
(Ragú):		
Regular	2 oz.	32
Pizza Quick	2 oz.	45
PLUM:		
Fresh, Japanese & hybrid	2″ dia.	27
Fresh, prune-type, halves	½ cup	60
Canned, regular pack:		
(Stokely-Van Camp)	½ cup	120
(Thank You Brand) heavy syrup	½ cup	109
Canned, unsweetened, purple, solids & liq.:		
(Diet Delight) juice pack	½ cup	70
(Featherweight) water pack	½ cup	40
(S&W) *Nutradiet,* juice pack	½ cup	80
PLUM JELLY, sweetened (Home Brands)	1 T.	52
PLUM PRESERVE OR JAM, sweetened (Bama)	1 T.	45
PLUM PUDDING (Richardson & Robbins)	2″ wedge	270
POLYNESIAN-STYLE DINNER, frozen (Swanson)	12-oz. dinner	360
POMEGRANATE, whole	1 lb.	160
PONDEROSA RESTAURANT:		
A-1 Sauce	1 tsp.	4
Beef, chopped (patty only):		
Regular	3½ oz.	209
Double Deluxe	5.9 oz.	362
Junior (*Square Shooter*)	1.6 oz.	98
Steakhouse Deluxe	2.96 oz.	181
Beverages:		
Coca-Cola	8 fl. oz.	96
Coffee	6 fl. oz.	2
Dr. Pepper	8 fl. oz.	96
Milk, chocolate	8 fl. oz.	208
Orange drink	8 fl. oz.	110
Root beer	8 fl. oz.	104
Sprite	8 fl. oz.	95
Tab	8 fl. oz.	1
Bun:		
Regular	2.4-oz. bun	190
Hot dog	1 bun	108
Junior	1.4-oz. bun	118
Steakhouse deluxe	2.4-oz. bun	190
Chicken strips:		
Adult portion	2¾ oz.	282
Child	1.4 oz.	141

Food and Description	Measure or Quantity	Calories
Cocktail sauce	1½ oz.	57
Filet mignon	3.8 oz. (edible portion)	57
Filet of sole, fish only (See also Bun, regular)	3-oz. piece	125
Fish, baked	4.9-oz. serving	268
Gelatin dessert	½ cup	97
Gravy, au jus	1 oz.	3
Ham & cheese:		
Bun (see Bun, regular)		
Cheese, Swiss	2 slices (.8 oz.)	76
Ham	2½ oz.	184
Hot dog, child's, meat only (see also Bun, junior)	1.6-oz. hot dog	140
Margarine:		
Pat	1 tsp.	36
On potato, as served	½ oz.	100
Mustard sauce, sweet & sour	1 oz.	50
New York strip steak	6.1 oz. (edible portion)	362
Onion, chopped	1 T.	4
Pickle, dill	3 slices (.7 oz.)	2
Potato:		
Baked	7.2-oz. potato	145
French fries	3-oz. serving	230
Prime ribs:		
Regular	4.2 oz. (edible portion)	286
King	6 oz. (edible portion)	409
Pudding, chocolate	4½ oz.	213
Ribeye	3.2 oz. (edible portion)	197
Ribeye & shrimp:		
Ribeye	3.2 oz.	197
Shrimp	2.2 oz.	139
Roll, kaiser	2.2-oz. roll	184
Salad bar:		
Bean sprouts	1 oz.	13
Broccoli	1 oz.	9
Cabbage, red	1 oz.	9
Carrots	1 oz.	12
Cauliflower	1 oz.	8
Celery	1 oz.	4
Chickpeas (Garbanzos)	1 oz.	102
Mushrooms	1 oz.	8
Pepper, green	1 oz.	6
Radish	1 oz.	5
Tomato	1 oz.	6

Food and Description	Measure or Quantity	Calories
Salad dressing:		
Blue cheese	1 oz.	129
Italian, creamy	1 oz.	138
Low calorie	1 oz.	14
Oil & vinegar	1 oz.	124
1000 Island	1 oz.	117
Shrimp dinner	7 pieces (3½ oz.)	220
Sirloin:		
Regular	3.3 oz. (edible portion)	220
Super	6½ oz. (edible portion)	383
Tips	4 oz. (edible portion)	192
Steak sauce	1 oz.	23
Tartar sauce	1.5 oz.	285
T-Bone	4.3 oz. (edible portion)	240
Tomato (See also Salad bar):		
Slices	2 slices (.9 oz.)	5
Whole, small	3.5 oz.	22
Topping, whipped	¼ oz.	19
Worcestershire sauce	1 tsp.	4
POPCORN:		
*Plain, popped fresh:		
(Jiffy Pop)	½ of 5-oz. pkg.	244
(Jolly Time) microwave:		
Natural or butter flavor	1 cup	53
Cheese flavor	1 cup	60
(Orville Reddenbacher's):		
Original:		
Plain	1 cup	22
With oil & salt	1 cup	40
Caramel crunch	1 oz.	140
Hot air popped	1 cup	25
Microwave:		
Regular:		
Butter flavored	1 cup	27
Natural	1 cup	27
Flavored:		
Caramel	1 cup	96
Cheese, cheddar	1 cup	50
Frozen	1 cup	35
(Pillsbury) microwave popcorn:		
Regular	1 cup	70
Butter flavor	1 cup	65
Pop Secret (General Mills)	1 cup	140
Packaged:		
Buttered (Wise)	½ oz.	70

Food and Description	Measure or Quantity	Calories
Caramel-coated:		
(Bachman)	1-oz. serving	130
(Old Dutch)	1 oz.	109
(Old London) without peanuts	1¾-oz. serving	195
Cheese flavored (Bachman)	1-oz. serving	180
Cracker Jack	1-oz. serving	120
POPCORN POPPING OIL (Orville Reddenbacher's) buttery flavor	1 T.	120
***POPOVER MIX** (Flako)	1 popover	170
POPPY SEED (French's)	1 tsp.	13
POPSICLE, twin pop	3 fl. oz.	70
POP TARTS (See TOASTER CAKE OR PASTRY)		
PORK:		
Fresh:		
Chop:		
Broiled, lean & fat	3-oz. chop (weighed without bone)	332
Broiled, lean only	3-oz. chop (weighed without bone)	230
Loin:		
Roasted, lean & fat	3 oz.	308
Roasted, lean only	3 oz.	216
Spareribs, braised	3 oz.	246
Cured ham:		
Roasted, lean & fat	3 oz.	246
Roasted, lean only	3 oz.	159
PORK DINNER OR ENTREE:		
Canned (Hunt's) *Minute Gourmet Microwave Entree Maker,* cajun:		
Without pork	3.9 oz.	180
*With pork	6.6 oz.	460
Frozen (Swanson) dinner, loin of	11¼-oz. dinner	290
PORK, PACKAGED (Eckrich)	1-oz. serving	45
PORK RINDS (Tom's)	.6 oz. serving	60
PORK STEAK, BREADED, frozen (Hormel)	3-oz. serving	223
PORK, SWEET & SOUR, frozen (La Choy)	½ of 15-oz. pkg.	229
PORT WINE:		
(Gallo)	3 fl. oz.	94
(Louis M. Martini)	3 fl. oz.	82
POSTUM, instant	6 fl. oz.	11
POTATO:		
Cooked:		
Au gratin	½ cup	127
Baked, peeled	2½"-dia. potato	92
Boiled, peeled	4.2-oz. potato	79
French-fried	10 pieces	156

Food and Description	Measure or Quantity	Calories
Hash-browned, home recipe	½ cup	223
Mashed, milk & butter added	½ cup	92
Canned, solids & liq.:		
(Allen's) *Butterfield*	½ cup	45
(Hunt's)	4 oz.	70
(Larsen) *Freshlike*, sliced or whole	½ cup (4.5 oz.)	61
Frozen:		
(Birds Eye):		
Cottage fries	2.8-oz. serving	119
Crinkle cuts, regular	3-oz. serving	115
Farm style wedge	3-oz. serving	109
French fries, regular	3-oz. serving	113
Hash browns, shredded	¼ of 12-oz. pkg.	61
Steak fries	3-oz. serving	109
Tasti Puffs	¼ of 10-oz. pkg.	192
Tiny Taters	⅓ of 16-oz. pkg.	204
Whole, peeled	3.2 oz.	59
(Empire Kosher) french fries	3 oz.	110
(Green Giant) one serving:		
Au gratin	5½ oz.	200
& broccoli	5½ oz.	130
(Larsen) diced	4 oz.	80
(Ore-Ida):		
Cheddar Browns	3 oz.	80
Cottage fries	3 oz.	120
Crispers!	3 oz.	230
Crispy Crowns	3 oz.	170
Golden Fries	3 oz.	120
Golden Patties	3 oz.	140
Hash browns:		
Microwave	2 oz.	120
Shredded	3 oz.	70
Toaster	1¾ oz.	100
Pixie crinkles	3 oz.	140
Shoestrings	3 oz.	150
Tater Tots:		
Plain, microwave	4 oz.	200
With bacon flavor	3 oz.	150
Whole, small, seeded	3 oz.	70
(Stouffer's):		
Au gratin	⅓ pkg.	110
Scalloped	⅓ pkg.	90
POTATO & BACON, canned		
(Hormel) *Short Orders*, au gratin	7½-oz. can	240
POTATO & BEEF, canned,		
Dinty Moore (Hormel) *Short Orders*	1½-oz. can	250
POTATO & HAM, canned (Hormel)		
Short Orders, scalloped	7½-oz. can	250

Food and Description	Measure or Quantity	Calories
POTATO CHIP:		
(Cape Cod) any flavor	1 oz.	150
(Cottage Fries) unsalted	1 oz.	160
Delta Gold, any style	1 oz.	160
(Eagle):		
All types except ridged, ranch	1 oz.	150
Ridged, ranch style	1 oz.	160
(Frito-Lay's) natural	1 oz.	157
Lay's, sour cream & onion flavor	1 oz.	160
(New York Deli)	1 oz.	160
O'Grady's	1 oz.	150
(Old Dutch):		
Regular or onion & garlic	1 oz.	150
BBQ	1 oz.	140
Pringle's:		
Regular or *Cheez-Ums*	1 oz.	167
Light	1 oz.	148
(Snyder's)	1 oz.	150
Ruffles, light	1 oz.	130
(Tom's) any type	1 oz.	160
(Wise):		
Barbecue or garlic & onion	1 oz.	150
Lightly salted, natural or salt & vinegar	1 oz.	160
***POTATO MIX:**		
Au gratin:		
(Betty Crocker)	½ cup	150
(French's) tangy	½ cup	130
(Lipton) & sauce	¼ pkg.	108
Casserole (French's)	½ cup	130
Cheddar bacon (Lipton) & sauce	½ cup	106
Cheddar broccoli (Lipton)	½ cup	104
Chicken flavored mushroom (Lipton) & sauce	¼ pkg.	90
Hash browns (Betty Crocker) with onion	½ cup	160
Italian (Lipton)	½ cup	107
Julienne (Betty Crocker) with mild cheese sauce	½ cup	130
Mashed:		
(Betty Crocker) *Buds*	½ cup	130
(French's)	½ cup	140
Nacho (Lipton) & sauce	½ cup	103
Scalloped:		
(Betty Crocker) plain	½ cup	140
(Libby's) *Potato Classics*	¾ cup	130
(Lipton) & sauce	¼ cup	102
*Smoky cheddar (Betty Crocker)	½ cup	140

Food and Description	Measure or Quantity	Calories
Sour cream & chive (Betty Crocker)	½ cup	160
Stroganoff (French's) creamy	½ cup	130
*POTATO PANCAKE MIX		
(French's)	3″ pancake	30
POTATO SALAD:		
Home recipe	½ cup	181
Canned (Nalley's) German style	4-oz. serving	143
*Mix, (Lipton) German	½ cup	99
POTATO STICKS (Durkee) *O & C*	1½-oz. can	231
POTATO, STUFFED, BAKED:		
*Mix (Betty Crocker):		
Bacon & cheese	⅙ pkg.	210
Cheddar, mild, with onion	⅙ pkg.	190
Sour cream & chive	⅙ pkg.	200
Frozen:		
(Ore-Ida):		
Butter flavor	5-oz. serving	210
Cheddar cheese	5-oz. serving	230
(Weight Watchers):		
Broccoli & cheese	10½-oz. pkg.	250
Chicken divan	11-oz. pkg.	270
POTATO TOPPERS (Libby's)	1 T.	30
POT ROAST, frozen:		
(Armour) *Dinner Classics,* yankee	10-oz. meal	310
(Healthy Choice) yankee	11-oz. meal	260
(Stouffer's) *Right Course*	9¼-oz. meal	220
POUND CAKE (See CAKE, Pound)		
PRESERVE OR JAM (See individual flavors)		
PRETZEL:		
(Eagle Snacks)	1 oz.	110
(Estee) unsalted	1 piece	7
Mister Salty:		
Regular:		
Dutch	.5-oz. piece	55
Logs	.1-oz. piece	12
Nuggets	1 piece	5
Rods	.5-oz. piece	55
Stick, *Veri-thin*	1 piece	2
(Rokeach)	1 oz.	110
Rold Gold	1 oz.	110
(Snyder's) hard	1 oz.	102
(Tom's) twists	1 oz.	100
(Wise) nugget	1 oz.	110
PRODUCT 19, cereal (Kellogg's)	1 cup (1 oz.)	100
PROSCIUTTO (Hormel) boneless	1 oz.	90
PRUNE:		
Canned:		
(Featherweight) stewed,		

Food and Description	Measure or Quantity	Calories
water pack	½ cup	130
(Sunsweet) stewed	½ cup	120
Dried:		
(Del Monte) Moist Pak	2 oz.	120
(Sunsweet) whole	2 oz.	130
PRUNE JUICE:		
(Algood) *Lady Betty*	6 fl. oz.	130
(Ardmore Farms)	6 fl. oz.	148
(Mott's)	6 fl. oz.	130
PRUNE NECTAR, canned (Mott's)	6 fl. oz.	100
PUDDING OR PIE FILLING:		
Canned, regular pack:		
Banana:		
(Del Monte) *Pudding Cup*	5-oz. container	181
(Hunt's) *Snack Pack*	4¼-oz. container	180
(Thank You Brand)	½ cup	150
Butterscotch:		
(Del Monte) *Pudding Cup*	5-oz. container	184
Swiss Miss	4-oz. container	160
(Thank You Brand)	½ cup	149
Chocolate:		
(Del Monte) *Pudding Cup*	5-oz. container	201
(Hunt's) *Snack Pack:*		
Regular	4¼-oz. container	160
Fudge	4¼-oz. container	170
Marshmallow	4¼-oz. container	190
Swiss Miss fudge or fruit on bottom	4-oz. container	170
(Thank You Brand)	½ cup	191
Rice (Comstock; Menner's)	½ of 7½-oz. can	120
Tapioca:		
(Del Monte) *Pudding Cup*	5-oz. container	172
(Hunt's) *Snack Pack*	4¼-oz. container	160
Vanilla (Del Monte)	5-oz. container	188
Canned, dietetic pack:		
(Estee)	½ cup	70
(Sego)	4-oz. serving	125
Chilled, *Swiss Miss:*		
Butterscotch, chocolate malt or vanilla	4-oz. container	150
Chocolate or double rich	4-oz. container	160
Tapioca	4-oz. container	130
Frozen (Rich's):		
Butterscotch	4½-oz. container	198
Chocolate	4½-oz. container	212
*Mix, sweetened, regular & instant:		
Banana:		
(Jell-O) cream, regular	½ cup	161
(Royal) regular	½ cup	160

Food and Description	Measure or Quantity	Calories
Butter pecan (Jello-O) instant	½ cup	175
Butterscotch:		
(Jell-O) instant	½ cup	175
(My-T-Fine) regular	½ cup	143
Chocolate		
(Jell-O) regular	½ cup	174
(My-T-Fine) regular	½ cup	169
Coconut:		
(Jell-O) cream, regular	½ cup	176
(Royal) instant	½ cup	170
Flan:		
(Knorr):		
Without sauce	½ cup	130
With sauce	½ cup	190
(Royal) regular	½ cup	150
Lemon:		
(Jell-O) instant	½ cup	170
(My-T-Fine) regular	½ cup	164
Lime (Royal) key lime, regular	½ cup	160
Pineapple (Jell-O) cream, instant	½ cup	176
Pistachio (Jell-O) instant	½ cup	174
Raspberry (Salada)		
Danish Dessert	½ cup	176
Rice, (Jell-O) *Americana*	½ cup	176
Strawberry (Salada)		
Danish Dessert	½ cup	130
Tapioca:		
(Jell-O) *Americana,* chocolate	½ cup	173
(My-T-Fine) vanilla	½ cup	130
Vanilla:		
(Jell-O) French, regular	½ cup	172
(Royal)	½ cup	180
*Mix, dietetic:		
Butterscotch:		
(D-Zerta)	½ cup	68
(Featherweight) artificially		
sweetened	½ cup	60
(Royal) instant	½ cup	100
(Weight Watchers)	½ cup	90
Chocolate:		
(Estee)	½ cup	70
(Royal) instant	½ cup	100
(Weight Watchers)	½ cup	90
Vanilla:		
(D-Zerta)	½ cup	71
(Estee)	½ cup	70
(Weight Watchers)	½ cup	90
PUDDING ROLL-UPS (General Mills) *Fruit Corners*	.5-oz. roll	60

Food and Description	Measure or Quantity	Calories
PUDDING STIX (Good Humor)	1¾-fl.-oz. pop	90
PUDDING SUNDAE *Swiss Miss*:		
Caramel or mint	4-oz. container	170
Chocolate	4-oz. container	190
Peanut butter	4-oz. container	200
PUFFED RICE:		
(Malt-O-Meal)	1 cup	54
(Quaker)	1 cup	55
PUFFED WHEAT:		
(Malt-O-Meal)	1 cup	53
(Quaker)	1 cup	54
PUMPKIN, canned (Libby's) solid pack	½ cup	80
PUMPKIN BUTTER (Smucker's) *Autumn Harvest*	1 T.	36
PUMPKIN SEED, in hull	1 oz.	116
PUNCH DRINK (Minute Maid):		
Canned:		
Concord, On the Go	10-fl.-oz. bottle	155
Tropical	8.45-fl.-oz. cont.	130
Chilled	6 fl. oz.	93
*Frozen, citrus	6 fl. oz.	93
PURE & LIGHT (Dole) canned:		
Country raspberry or mountain cherry	6 fl. oz.	90
Mandarin orange	6 fl. oz.	100

Q

Food and Description	Measure or Quantity	Calories
QUAIL, raw, meat & skin	4 oz.	195
QUIK, (Nestlé):		
Regular, chocolate or strawberry	1 tsp.	45
Sugar free	1 tsp.	18
QUISP, cereal	1⅙ cup	121

R

Food and Description	Measure or Quantity	Calories
RADISH	2 small radishes	4
RAISIN, dried:		
(Dole)	¼ cup	125
(Sun-Maid)	1 oz.	96
RAISIN SQUARES, cereal		
(Kellogg's)	½ cup	90
RALSTON, cereal (Ralston Purina)	¼ cup	90
RASPBERRY:		
Fresh:		
Black, trimmed	½ cup	49
Red, trimmed	½ cup	41
Frozen (Birds Eye) quick thaw	5-oz. serving	155
*****RASPBERRY DRINK,** mix		
(Funny Face)	8 fl. oz.	88
RASPBERRY PRESERVE OR JAM:		
Sweetened (Smucker's)	1 T.	54
Dietetic:		
(Estee, Louis Sherry)	1 T.	6
(Slenderella)	1 T.	21
(S&W) *Nutradiet,* red	1 T.	12
RATATOUILLE, frozen (Stouffer's)	5-oz. serving	60
RAVIOLI:		
Canned, regular		
(Franco-American) beef,		
RavioliOs	7½-oz. serving	210
Canned, dietetic (Estee) beef	8-oz. can	230
Frozen:		
(Buitoni):		
Cheese:		
Regular, square	4.8 oz.	331
Ravioletti	2.6 oz.	221
Meat, square	4.8 oz.	318
(Celentano):		
Regular	6½ oz.	380
Mini	4 oz.	250
(Kid Cuisine) cheese, mini	8¾-oz. pkg.	250
(Weight Watchers) baked	9 oz. meal	290

Food and Description	Measure or Quantity	Calories
RED LOBSTER RESTAURANT		
("Lunch portion" refers to a cooked serving weighing 5 oz. raw, unless otherwise noted):		
Calamari, breaded & fried	Lunch portion	360
Catfish	Lunch portion	170
Chicken breast	4-oz. serving	120
Clam, cherrystone	Lunch portion	130
Cod, Atlantic	Lunch portion	100
Crab legs:		
King	16-oz. serving	170
Snow	16-oz. serving	150
Flounder	Lunch portion	100
Grouper	Lunch portion	110
Haddock	Lunch portion	100
Halibut	Lunch portion	110
Hamburger, without bun	5.3 oz.	320
Lobster:		
Maine	1 lobster (edible portion)	240
Rock	1 tail	230
Mackerel	Lunch portion	190
Monkfish	Lunch portion	110
Mussels	3-oz. serving	70
Oysters	6 raw oysters	110
Perch, Atlantic Ocean	Lunch portion	130
Pollock	Lunch portion	120
Rockfish, red	Lunch portion	90
Salmon:		
Norwegian	Lunch portion	230
Sockeye	Lunch portion	160
Scallop:		
Calico	Lunch portion	180
Deep sea	Lunch portion	130
Shark:		
Blacktip	Lunch portion	150
Mako	Lunch portion	140
Shrimp	8–12 pieces	120
Snapper, red	Lunch portion	110
Sole, lemon	Lunch portion	120
Steak:		
Porterhouse	18-oz. serving	1420
Sirloin	7-oz. serving	570
Strip	7-oz. serving	690
Swordfish	Lunch portion	100
Tilefish	Lunch portion	100
Trout, rainbow	Lunch portion	170
Tuna, yellowfin	Lunch portion	180

Food and Description	Measure or Quantity	Calories
RELISH:		
Dill (Vlasic)	1 oz.	2
Hamburger:		
(Heinz)	1 oz.	30
(Vlasic)	1 T.	24
Hot dog:		
(Heinz)	1 oz.	35
(Vlasic)	1 T.	28
Sweet (Vlasic)	1 T.	18
RENNET MIX (Junket):		
*Powder, any flavor:		
Made with skim milk	½ cup	90
Made with whole milk	½ cup	120
Tablet	1 tablet	1
RHINE WINE:		
(Great Western)	3 fl. oz.	73
(Taylor)	3 fl. oz.	75
RHUBARB, cooked, sweetened	½ cup	169
***RICE:**		
Brown (Uncle Ben's) parboiled, with added butter	⅔ cup	152
White:		
(Minute Rice) instant, no added butter	⅔ cup	120
(Success) long grain	½ cooking bag	110
White & wild (Carolina)	½ cup	90
RICE CAKE:		
(Hain):		
Regular	1 piece	40
Mini:		
Plain, apple cinnamon or teriyaki	½-oz. serving	50
Barbecue or nacho cheese	½-oz. serving	70
Cheese or honey nut	½-oz. serving	60
Heart Lovers (TKI Foods) lightly salted	.3-oz. piece	35
(Pritikin)	1 piece	35
RICE, FRIED (See also RICE MIX):		
*Canned (La Choy)	¾ cup	180
Frozen:		
(Birds Eye)	3.7-oz. serving	104
(Chun King) pork—	8 oz.	270
(La Choy) & meat	8-oz. serving	280
RICE, FRIED, SEASONING MIX (Kikkoman)	1-oz. pkg.	91
***RICE KRINKLES,** cereal (Post)	⅞ cup	109
***RICE KRISPIES,** cereal (Kellogg's):		
Regular, frosted, cocoa or strawberry	1 oz.	110
Marshmallow	1 oz.	140

Food and Description	Measure or Quantity	Calories
RICE MIX:		
Beef:		
*(Carolina) *Bake-It-Easy*	¼ pkg.	110
(Lipton) & sauce	¼ pkg.	120
*(Minute Rice)	½ cup	149
Rice-A-Roni	⅙ pkg.	130
*Cajun (Lipton) & sauce	¼ pkg.	123
Chicken:		
*(Carolina) *Bake-It-Easy*	¼ pkg.	110
(Lipton) & sauce	¼ pkg.	125
Rice-A-Roni	⅙ pkg.	130
*Fried (Minute Rice)	½ cup	160
Herb & butter (Lipton) & sauce	¼ pkg.	124
*Long grain & wild (Minute Rice)	½ cup	150
*Milanese (Knorr) risotto, with saffron	½ cup	130
Mushroom (Lipton) & sauce	¼ pkg.	123
*Oriental (Carolina) *Bake-It-Easy*	½ pkg.	120
*Pilaf (Lipton) & sauce	½ cup	117
Spanish:		
*(Carolina) *Bake-It-Easy*	¼ pkg.	110
*(Lipton) & sauce	½ cup	120
Rice-A-Roni	⅐ pkg.	110
*Tomato (Knorr) risotto	½ cup	130
*RICE SEASONING (French's)		
Spice Your Rice:		
Beef flavor & onion or cheese & chives	½ cup	160
Buttery herb	½ cup	170
RICE, SPANISH:		
Canned:		
Regular pack (Comstock; Menner's)	½ of 7½-oz. can	140
Dietetic (Featherweight) low sodium	7½-oz. serving	140
Frozen (Birds Eye)	3.7-oz. serving	122
RICE & VEGETABLE:		
*Mix:		
(Knorr) risotto	½ cup	130
(Lipton) & sauce:		
& asparagus with Hollandaise sauce	½ cup	123
& broccoli with cheddar	½ cup	131
Frozen:		
(Birds Eye):		
For One:		
& broccoli, au gratin	5¾-oz. pkg.	229
Mexican, with corn	5½-oz. pkg.	158
pilaf	5½-oz. pkg.	215

Food and Description	Measure or Quantity	Calories
Internationals:		
Country style	3.3 oz.	87
Spanish style	3.3 oz.	111
(Green Giant):		
One Serving:		
& broccoli in cheese sauce	4½-oz. pkg.	180
With peas & mushrooms with sauce	5½-oz. pkg.	130
Rice Originals:		
Medley	½ cup	100
Pilaf	½ cup	110
& wild rice	½ cup	130
RICE WINE:		
Chinese, 20.7% alcohol	1 fl. oz.	38
Japanese, 10.6% alcohol	1 fl. oz.	72
RIGATONI, frozen		
(Healthy Choice) & meat sauce	9½-oz. meal	240
ROCK & RYE (Mr. Boston)	1 fl. oz.	75
ROCKY ROAD, cereal (General Mills)	⅔ cup (1 oz.)	120
ROE, baked or broiled, cod & shad	4 oz.	143
ROLL OR BUN:		
Commercial type, non-frozen:		
Apple (Dolly Madison)	2-oz. piece	180
Biscuit (Wonder)	1¼-oz. piece	80
Brown & serve:		
Merita (Interstate Brands)	1-oz. roll	70
(Roman Meal) original	1-oz. roll	72
Cherry (Dolly Madison)	2-oz. piece	180
Cinnamon (Dolly Madison)	1¾-oz. piece	180
Club (Pepperidge Farm)	1.3-oz. piece	100
Crescent (Pepperidge Farm) butter	1-oz. piece	110
Croissant (Pepperidge Farm):		
Butter, cinnamon or honey-sesame	2-oz. piece	200
Chocolate	2.4-oz. piece	260
Walnut	2-oz. piece	210
Danish (Dolly Madison)		
Danish Twirls:		
Apple	2-oz. piece	240
Cheese, cream	3½-oz. piece	380
Cinnamon raisin	2-oz. piece	250
Dinner:		
Butternut (Interstate Brands)	1-oz. roll	90
Home Pride	1-oz. piece	85
(Pepperidge Farm)	.7-oz. piece	60
(Roman Meal)	1-oz. roll	75
Finger (Pepperidge Farm) sesame or poppy seed	.6-oz. piece	60

Food and Description	Measure or Quantity	Calories
Frankfurter:		
(Arnold) Hot Dog	1.3-oz. piece	100
(Pepperidge Farm)	1¾-oz. piece	110
(Roman Meal)	1.5-oz. roll	114
French:		
(Arnold) *Francisco*, sourdough	1.1-oz. piece	90
(Pepperidge Farm):		
Small	1.3-oz. piece	110
Large	3-oz. piece	240
Golden Twist (Pepperidge Farm)	1-oz. piece	110
Hamburger:		
(Arnold)	1.4-oz. piece	110
(Pepperidge Farm)	1.5-oz. piece	130
(Roman Meal)	1.6-oz. piece	122
Hoagie (Wonder)	5-oz. piece	400
Honey (Dolly Madison)	3½-oz. piece	420
Kaiser (Interstate Brands):		
Dutch Hearth	1½-oz. piece	110
Sweetheart	2-oz. piece	150
Lemon (Dolly Madison)	2-oz. piece	180
Old fashioned (Pepperidge Farm)	.6-oz. piece	60
Parkerhouse (Pepperidge Farm)	.6-oz. piece	50
Party (Pepperidge Farm)	.4-oz. piece	30
Raspberry (Dolly Madison)	2-oz. piece	190
Sandwich (Arnold) soft	1.3-oz. piece	110
Soft (Pepperidge Farm)	1¼-oz. piece	110
*ROLL OR BUN DOUGH:		
Frozen (Rich's) home style	1 piece	75
Refrigerated (Pillsbury):		
Caramel danish, with nuts	1 piece	160
Cinnamon raisin danish	1 piece	110
Crescent	1 piece	100
*ROLL MIX, HOT (Pillsbury)	1 piece	120
ROMAN MEAL CEREAL, hot:		
Regular:		
Cream of rye	⅓ cup (1.3 oz.)	112
Oat bran		
Oat, wheat, dates, raisins, almonds	⅓ cup	136
Original, plain	⅓ cup (1 oz.)	82
Instant, oats, wheat, honey, coconut, almond	⅓ cup	154
ROSEMARY LEAVES (French's)	1 tsp.	5
ROSÉ WINE:		
Corbett Canyon (Glenmore)	3 fl. oz.	63
(Great Western)	3 fl. oz.	80
(Paul Masson):		
Regular, 11.8% alcohol	3 fl. oz.	76
Light, 7.1% alcohol	3 fl. oz.	49

Food and Description	Measure or Quantity	Calories
ROY ROGERS RESTAURANTS:		
Bar Burger	1 serving	573
Biscuit	1 biscuit	231
Breakfast crescent sandwich:		
Regular	4.5-oz. sandwich	408
With bacon	4.7-oz. sandwich	446
With ham	5.8-oz. sandwich	456
With sausage	5.7-oz. sandwich	564
Cheeseburger:		
Regular	1 serving	525
With bacon	1 serving	552
Chicken:		
Breast	1 piece	412
Leg	1 piece	140
Thigh	1 piece	296
Wing	1 piece	192
Chicken nugget	1 piece	48
Coleslaw	3½-oz. serving	110
Drinks:		
Coffee, black	6 fl. oz.	Tr.
Coke:		
Regular	12 fl. oz.	145
Diet	12 fl. oz.	1
Hot chocolate	6 fl. oz.	123
Milk	8 fl. oz.	150
Orange juice:		
Regular	7 fl. oz.	99
Large	10 fl. oz.	136
Shake:		
Chocolate	1 shake	358
Strawberry	1 shake	306
Vanilla	1 shake	315
Tea, iced, plain	8 fl. oz.	0
Egg & biscuit platter:		
Regular	1 meal (5.8 oz.)	557
With bacon	1 meal (6.1 oz.)	607
With ham	1 meal (7 oz.)	605
With sausage	1 meal (7.2 oz.)	713
Hamburger	1 burger	472
Pancake platter, with syrup & butter		
Plain	1 order	386
With bacon	1 order	436
With ham	1 order	434
With sausage	1 order	542
Potato french fries:		
Regular	4 oz.	320
Large	5.5 oz.	440
Potato salad	3½-oz. order	107

Food and Description	Measure or Quantity	Calories
Roast beef sandwich:		
Plain:		
Regular	1 sandwich	350
Large	1 sandwich	373
With cheese:		
Regular	1 sandwich	403
Large	1 sandwich	427
Salad bar:		
Bacon bits	1 T.	33
Beets, sliced	¼ cup	18
Broccoli	½ cup	12
Carrot, shredded	¼ cup	12
Cheese, cheddar	¼ cup	112
Croutons	1 T.	35
Egg, chopped	1 T.	27
Lettuce	1 cup	10
Macaroni salad	1 T.	30
Mushrooms	¼ cup	5
Noodles, Chinese	¼ cup	55
Pepper, green	1 T.	2
Potato salad	1 T.	25
Tomato	1 slice	7
Salad dressing:		
Regular:		
Bacon & tomato	1 T.	68
Bleu cheese	1 T.	75
Ranch	1 T.	77
1000 Island	1 T.	80
Low calorie, Italian	1 T.	35
Strawberry shortcake	7.2-oz. serving	447
Sundae:		
Caramel	1 sundae	293
Hot fudge	1 sundae	337
Strawberry	1 sundae	216
RUM (See DISTILLED LIQUOR)		
RUTABAGA:		
Canned (Sunshine) solids & liq.	½ cup	32
Frozen (Sunshine)	4 oz.	50

S

Food and Description	Measure or Quantity	Calories
SAFFLOWER SEED, in hull	1 oz.	89
SAGE (French's)	1 tsp.	4
SAKE WINE	1 fl. oz.	39
SALAD CRUNCHIES (Libby's)	1 T.	35
SALAD DRESSING:		
Regular:		
Bacon (Seven Seas) creamy	1 T.	60
Bacon & tomato (Henri's)	1 T.	70
Bleu or blue cheese		
(Henri's)	1 T.	60
Buttermilk (Hain)	1 T.	70
Caesar:		
(Hain)	1 T.	60
(Pfeiffer)	1 T.	70
(Wish-Bone)	1 T.	78
Capri (Seven Seas)	1 T.	70
Cheddar & bacon (Wish-Bone)	1 T.	70
Cucumber (Wish-Bone)	1 T.	80
Dijon vinaigrette (Hain)	1 T.	50
French:		
(Hain) creamy	1 T.	60
(Henri's):		
Hearty	1 T.	70
Original	1 T.	60
(Wish-Bone) garlic	1 T.	55
Garlic (Wish-Bone) creamy	1 T.	74
Garlic & sour cream (Hain)	1 T.	70
Green Goddess (Seven Seas)	1 T.	60
Honey & sesame (Hain)	1 T.	60
Italian:		
(Hain):		
Canola oil	1 T.	50
Creamy or traditional	1 T.	80
(Henri's):		
Authentic	1 T.	80
Creamy garlic	1 T.	50
(Pfeiffer) chef	1 T.	60
(Seven Seas) *Viva!*	1 T.	70

Food and Description	Measure or Quantity	Calories
(Wish-Bone) robusto	1 T.	70
Mayonnaise-type		
(Luzianne Blue Plate)	1 T.	70
Miracle Whip (Kraft)	1 T.	70
Poppyseed rancher's (Hain)	1 T.	60
Ranch (Henri's) *Chef's Recipe*	1 T.	70
Red wine vinegar & oil		
(Seven Seas)	1 T.	60
Roquefort:		
(Bernstein's)	1 T.	65
(Marie's)	1 T.	105
Russian:		
(Henri's)	1 T.	60
(Pfeiffer)	1 T.	65
(Wish-Bone)	1 T.	47
Sour cream & bacon (Wish-Bone)	1 T.	70
Spin Blend (Hellmann's)	1 T.	57
Swiss cheese vinaigrette (Hain)	1 T.	60
Tangy citrus (Hain)	1 T.	50
Tas-Tee (Henri's)	1 T.	60
Thousand Island:		
(Pfeiffer)	1 T.	65
(Wish-Bone) plain	1 T.	61
Vinaigrette (Bernstein's) french	1 T.	49
Dietetic or low calorie:		
Bleu or blue cheese:		
(Estee)	1 T.	8
(Featherweight) imitation	1 T.	4
(Henri's)	1 T.	35
(Tillie Lewis) *Tasti-Diet*	1 T.	12
(Walden Farms) chunky	1 T.	27
(Wish-Bone) chunky	1 T.	40
Caesar:		
(Hain) creamy, low salt	1 T.	60
(Weight Watchers)	¾-oz. pouch	6
Catalina (Kraft)	1 T.	16
Chef's Recipe Ranchouse (Henri's)	1 T.	40
Cucumber (Kraft)	1 T.	30
Dijon (Estee) creamy	1 T.	8
French:		
(Estee)	1 T.	4
(Henri's) original	1 T.	40
(Pritikin)	1 T.	10
(Wish-Bone)	1 T.	31
Herb basket, *Herb Magic*		
(Luzianne Blue Plate)	1 T.	6
Herb & spice (Featherweight)	1 T.	6
Garlic (Estee)	1 T.	2
Italian:		
(Estee) creamy	1 T.	4

Food and Description	Measure or Quantity	Calories
(Hain) no added salt, creamy	1 T.	80
(Henri's) hearty	1 T.	35
Herb Magic (Luzianne Blue Plate)	1 T.	4
(Pritikin) creamy	1 T.	16
(Weight Watchers) regular	1 T.	50
(Wish-Bone)	1 T.	7
Olive oil vinaigrette (Wish-Bone)	1 T.	16
Onion & chive (Wish-Bone)	1 T.	37
Ranch (Pritikin)	1 T.	18
Red wine/vinegar (Featherweight)	1 T.	6
Russian:		
(Pritikin)	1 T.	12
(Weight Watchers)	1 T.	50
(Wish-Bone)	1 T.	25
Sweet & sour, *Herb Magic* (Luzianne Blue Plate)	1 T.	18
Tas-Tee (Henri's)	1 T.	30
Thousand Island:		
(Estee)	1 T.	8
(Henri's)	1 T.	30
Herb Magic (Luzianne Blue Plate)	1 T.	8
(Kraft)	1 T.	30
(Walden Farms)	1 T.	24
(Weight Watchers)	1 T.	50
(Wish-Bone)	1 T.	40
Tomato (Pritikin) zesty	1 T.	18
2-Calorie Low Sodium (Featherweight)	1 T.	2
Vinaigrette (Pritikin)	1 T.	10
Whipped (Weight Watchers)	1 T.	45
SALAD DRESSING MIX:		
*Regular (Good Seasons):		
Blue cheese & herbs	1 T.	72
Buttermilk, farm style	1 T.	58
Garlic, cheese	1 T.	72
Garlic & herb	1 T.	71
Italian, regular, cheese or zesty	1 T.	71
*Dietetic:		
Bleu cheese (Hain) no oil	1 T.	14
Buttermilk (Hain) no oil	1 T.	11
Caesar (Hain) no oil	1 T.	6
French (Hain) no oil	1 T.	12
Italian:		
(Good Seasons) lite, zesty	1 T.	26
(Hain) no oil	1 T.	2
Ranch (Good Seasons) lite	1 T.	29
1000 Island (Hain) no oil	1 T.	12

Food and Description	Measure or Quantity	Calories
SALAD SUPREME (McCormick)	1 tsp.	11
SALAMI:		
(Eckrich) beer or cooked	1 oz.	70
Hebrew National, beef	1 oz.	80
(Hormel):		
Beef	1 slice	40
Genoa, DiLusso	1-oz. serving	100
Hard, sliced	1 slice	34
(Ohse) cooked	1 oz.	65
(Oscar Mayer):		
Beer, beef	.8-oz. slice	64
Cotto	.8-oz. slice	53
Genoa	.3-oz. slice	34
SALISBURY STEAK, frozen:		
(Armour) *Classics Lite*	11½-oz. meal	300
(Banquet) dinner:		
Regular	11-oz. meal	500
Extra Helping	18-oz. meal	910
(Healthy Choice)	11½-oz. meal	300
(Morton)	10-oz. meal	300
(Stouffer's) *Lean Cuisine*	9½-oz. pkg.	280
(Swanson):		
Regular:		
Dinner, 4-compartment	11-oz. dinner	460
Entree	5½-oz. entree	370
Hungry Man	16½-oz. dinner	710
Main Course	8½-oz. entree	430
(Weight Watchers) beef, Romano	8¾-oz. meal	310
SALMON:		
Baked or broiled	(5.1 oz.)	264
Canned, regular pack, solids & liq.:		
Chum, *Humpty Dumpty*		
(Peter Pan) Alaska	½ cup	140
Keta (Bumble Bee)	½ cup	153
Pink or Humpback:		
(Demings) skinless & boneless	2 oz.	80
(Double "Q")	½ of 6½-oz. can	120
(Peter Pan)	½ cup	140
Sockeye or Red or Blueback:		
(Double "Q") red sockeye	½ cup	170
(Gil Netters Best) blueback	½ cup	170
Canned, dietetic (S&W) *Nutradiet,* low sodium	½ cup	188
SALMON, SMOKED (Vita):		
Lox, drained	4-oz. jar	136
Nova, drained	4-oz. can	221
SALT:		
Regular & iodized (Morton):		
Regular	1 tsp.	0

Food and Description	Measure or Quantity	Calories
Lite	1 tsp.	0
Substitute:		
(Adolph's) plain	1 tsp.	1
Happy Heart (TKI Foods)		
Just Like Salt	¾-oz. packet	<1
(Morton) plain	1 tsp.	Tr.
Salt-It (Estee)	1 tsp.	0
SALT 'N SPICE SEASONING		
(McCormick)	1 tsp.	3
SANDWICH SPREAD:		
(Hellmann's)	1 T.	65
(Oscar Mayer)	1-oz. serving	67
SANGRIA (Taylor)	3 fl. oz.	99
SARDINE, canned:		
Atlantic (Del Monte) with		
tomato sauce	7½-oz. can	319
Imported (Underwood) in mustard		
or tomato sauce	3¾-oz. can	220
Norwegian:		
(Granadaisa Brand) in tomato sauce	3¾-oz. can	195
(King David Brand) brisling in		
olive oil	3¾-oz. can	293
(Queen Helga Brand) in sild oil	3¾-oz. can	310
SAUCE:		
Regular:		
A-1	1 T.	12
Barbecue:		
(Heinz)	¼ cup	80
(Hunt's)	1 T.	20
(Kraft) plain or hot	¼ cup	80
(La Choy) oriental	1 T.	16
Burrito (Del Monte)	¼ cup	20
Caramel (Knorr)	1 T.	60
Cheese (Snow's) welsh rarebit	½ cup	170
Chili (See CHILI SAUCE)		
Cocktail:		
(Gold's)	1 T.	31
(Pfeiffer)	1-oz. serving	100
Escoffier Sauce Diable	1 T.	20
Escoffier Sauce Robert	1 T.	20
Grilling & broiling (Knorr):		
Chardonnay	⅛ pkg.	50
Spicy plum	⅛ pkg.	60
Tuscan herb	⅛ pkg.	55
Hollandaise (Knorr) microwave	1/12 pkg.	50
Hot (Gebhardt)	1 tsp.	0
Italian (See also SPAGHETTI		
SAUCE or TOMATO SAUCE):		
(Contadina)	4-oz. serving	71

Food and Description	Measure or Quantity	Calories
(Ragú) red cooking	3½-oz. serving	45
Mandarin ginger (Knorr) microwave	⅛ pkg.	55
Newberg (Snow's)	⅓ cup	120
Orange (La Choy)	1 T.	23
Parmesano (Knorr) microwave	⅛ pkg.	50
Plum (La Choy) tangy	1 oz.	44
Salsa Brava (La Victoria)	1 T.	6
Salsa Casero (La Victoria)	1 T.	4
Salsa Jalapeño (La Victoria)	1 T.	4
Salsa Mexicana (Contadina)	4 fl. oz.	38
Salsa Picante (La Victoria)	1 T.	4
Salsa Ranchero (La Victoria)	1 T.	6
Salsa Roja (Del Monte)	¼ cup	20
Salsa Suprema (La Victoria)	1 T.	4
Seafood cocktail (Del Monte)	1 T.	21
Soy:		
(Chun King)	1 T.	5
(Gold's)	1 T.	10
(Kikkoman) light	1 T.	13
(La Choy)	1 T.	Tr.
Spare rib (Gold's)	1 oz.	60
Sweet & sour:		
(Chun King)	1.8 oz.	57
(Contadina)	4 fl. oz.	150
(La Choy)	1 T.	30
Szechuan (La Choy) hot & spicy	1 oz.	48
Tabasco	¼ tsp.	Tr.
Taco:		
(La Victoria) red	1 T.	6
(Old El Paso) hot or mild	1 T.	5
(Ortega) hot or mild	1 oz.	13
Tartar:		
(Hellmann's)	1 T.	73
(Nalley's)	1 T.	89
Teriyaki (Kikkoman)	1 T.	15
V-8	1-oz. serving	25
Vera cruz (Knorr) microwave	¼ pkg.	65
White, medium	¼ cup	103
Worcestershire:		
(French's) regular or smoky	1 T.	10
(Gold's)	1 T.	42
Dietetic:		
Barbecue (Estee)	1 T.	18
Mexican (Pritikin)	1 oz.	12
Soy:		
(Kikkoman)	1 T.	9
(La Choy)	1 T.	<1

Food and Description	Measure or Quantity	Calories
Steak (Estee)	½ oz.	14
Tartar (Weight Watchers)	1 T.	35
SAUCE MIX, regular:		
À la King (Durkee)	1-oz. pkg.	133
*Au jus (Knorr)	2 fl. oz.	8
*Bernaise (Knorr)	2 fl. oz.	170
*Cheese:		
(Durkee)	½ cup	168
(French's)	½ cup	160
*Demi-glace (Knorr)	2 fl. oz.	30
Hollandaise:		
(Durkee)	1-oz. pkg.	173
*(French's)	1 T.	15
*(Knorr)	2 fl. oz.	170
*Hunter (Knorr)	2 fl. oz.	25
*Italian (Knorr) Napoli	4 fl. oz.	100
*Lyonnaise (Knorr)	2 fl. oz.	20
*Mushroom (Knorr)	2 fl. oz.	60
*Pepper (Knorr)	2 fl. oz.	20
*Sweet & sour (Kikkoman)	1 T.	18
SAUERKRAUT, canned:		
(Claussen) drained	½ cup	16
(Comstock) regular	½ cup	30
(Frank's) Bavarian	½ cup	64
(Silver Floss) solids & liq.:		
Regular	½ cup	30
Krispy Kraut	½ cup	25
(Vlasic)	2 oz.	8
SAUSAGE:		
*Brown & Serve (Hormel)	1 sausage	70
Links (Ohse) hot	1 oz.	80
Patty (Hormel)	1 patty	150
Polish-style:		
(Eckrich)	1-oz. serving	95
(Hormel) *Kilbase*	1-oz. serving	122
(Ohse) regular	1 oz.	80
Pork:		
(Eckrich)	1-oz. link	100
*(Hormel) *Little Sizzlers*	1 link	51
(Jimmy Dean)	2-oz. serving	227
*(Oscar Mayer) *Little Friers*	1 link	79
Roll (Eckrich) minced	1-oz. slice	80
Smoked:		
(Eckrich) beef, *Smok-Y-Links*	.8-oz. link	70
(Hormel) smokies	1 sausage	80
(Ohse)	1 oz.	80
(Oscar Mayer) beef	1½-oz. link	126
*Turkey (Louis Rich) links or tube	1-oz. serving	45

Food and Description	Measure or Quantity	Calories
Vienna:		
(Hormel) regular	1 sausage	50
(Libby's) in barbecue sauce	2½-oz. serving	180
SAUTERNE:		
(Great Western)	3 fl. oz.	79
(Taylor)	3 fl. oz.	81
SCALLOP:		
Steamed	4-oz. serving	127
Frozen:		
(Mrs. Paul's) breaded & fried	3½-oz. serving	210
(Stouffer's) *Lean Cuisine*	11-oz. pkg.	230
SCHNAPPS, APPLE (Mr. Boston)	1 fl. oz.	78
SCHNAPPS, PEPPERMINT		
(Mr. Boston)	1 fl. oz.	115
SCOTCH (See DISTILLED LIQUOR)		
SCREWDRIVER COCKTAIL		
(Mr. Boston) 12½% alcohol	3 fl. oz.	111
SCROD DINNER OR ENTREE,		
frozen (Gorton's) microwave	1 pkg.	320
SEAFOOD NEWBURG, frozen:		
(Armour) *Dinner Classics*	11½-oz. meal	300
(Mrs. Paul's)	8½ oz.	310
SEAFOOD PLATTER, frozen		
(Mrs. Paul's) breaded & fried	9-oz. serving	510
SEGO DIET FOOD, canned:		
Regular	10-fl.-oz. can	225
Lite	10-fl.-oz. can	150
SELTZER (Canada Dry)	Any quantity	0
SERUTAN	1 tsp.	6
SESAME SEEDS (French's)	1 tsp.	9
7-GRAIN CEREAL		
(Loma Linda)	1 oz.	110
SHAD, CREOLE, home recipe	4-oz. serving	172
SHAKE 'N BAKE:		
Chicken:		
Original recipe	5½-oz. pkg.	617
Barbecue	7-oz. pkg.	741
Fish, original recipe	4.2-oz. pkg.	482
Pork or ribs:		
Original recipe	6-oz. pkg.	652
Extra crispy, *Oven Fry*	4.2-oz. pkg.	482
SHAKEY'S RESTAURANT:		
Chicken, fried, & potatoes:		
3-piece	1 order	947
5-piece	1 order	1700
Ham & cheese sandwich	1 sandwich	550
Pizza:		
Cheese:		
Thin	13″ pizza	1403

Food and Description	Measure or Quantity	Calories
Thick	13″ pizza	1890
Onion, green pepper, olive & mushroom:		
Thin	13″ pizza	1713
Thick	13″ pizza	2200
Pepperoni:		
Thin	13″ pizza	1833
Thick	13″ pizza	2320
Sausage & mushroom:		
Thin	13″ pizza	1759
Thick	13″ pizza	2256
Sausage & pepperoni:		
Thin	13″ pizza	2111
Thick	13″ pizza	2598
Special:		
Thin	13″ pizza	2110
Thick	13″ pizza	2597
Potatoes	15-piece order	950
Spaghetti with meat sauce & garlic bread	1 order	940
Super hot hero	1 sandwich	810
SHARK BITES (General Mills) *Fruit Corners*	.9-oz. pouch	100
SHELLS, PASTA, STUFFED, frozen:		
(Buitoni) jumbo, cheese stuffed	5½-oz. serving	288
(Celentano):		
Broccoli & cheese	13.5-oz. pkg.	540
Cheese:		
Without sauce	½ of 12½-oz. pkg.	350
With sauce	½ of 16-oz. pkg.	320
(Stouffer's) cheese stuffed	9-oz. serving	320
SHERBET OR SORBET:		
Lemon (Häagen-Dazs)	4 fl. oz.	140
Orange:		
(Baskin-Robbins)	4 fl. oz.	158
(Borden)	½ cup	110
(Dole) mandarin	½ cup	110
(Häagen-Dazs)	4 fl. oz.	113
Peach (Dole)	½ cup	130
Pineapple (Dole)	½ cup	120
Rainbow (Baskin-Robbins)	4 fl. oz.	160
Raspberry:		
(Baskin-Robbins)	4 fl. oz.	140
(Dole)	½ cup	110
(Häagen-Dazs)	4 fl. oz.	93
(Sealtest)	½ cup	140
SHERBET OR SORBET & ICE CREAM (Häagen-Dazs):		
Bar, orange & cream	1 bar	130

Food and Description	Measure or Quantity	Calories
Bulk:		
Blueberry, key lime or orange & cream	4 fl. oz.	190
Raspberry & cream	4 fl. oz.	180
SHERBET SHAKE, mix		
(Weight Watchers) orange	1 envelope	70
SHERRY:		
Cocktail (Gold Seal)	3 fl. oz.	122
Cream (Great Western) Solera	3 fl. oz.	141
Dry (Williams & Humbert)	3 fl. oz.	120
Dry Sack (Williams & Humbert)	3 fl. oz.	120
SHORTENING (See FAT, COOKING)		
SHREDDED WHEAT:		
(Kellogg's) *Squares*	½ cup (1 oz.)	90
(Nabisco):		
Regular size	¾-oz. biscuit	90
Spoon Size	⅔ cup	110
(Quaker)	1 biscuit	52
(Sunshine):		
Regular	1 biscuit	90
Bite size	⅔ cup	110
SHRIMP:		
Canned (Bumble Bee) solids & liq.	4½-oz. can	90
Frozen (Mrs. Paul's):		
Breaded & fried	3 oz.	190
Parmesan	11-oz. meal	310
SHRIMP & CHICKEN CANTONESE, frozen (Stouffer's) with noodles	10⅛-oz. meal	270
SHRIMP COCKTAIL canned or frozen (Sau-Sea)	4 oz.	113
SHRIMP DINNER, frozen:		
(Armour) *Classics Lite,* baby	9¾-oz. meal	220
(Gorton's) scampi, microwave entree	1 pkg.	470
(Healthy Choice) creole	11¼-oz. meal	210
(La Choy) Fresh & Lite, with lobster sauce	10-oz. meal	240
(Stouffer's) *Right Course,* primavera	9⅝-oz meal	240
SLENDER (Carnation):		
Bar	1 bar	135
Dry	1 packet	110
Liquid	10-fl.-oz. can	220
SLOPPY JOE:		
Canned:		
(Hormel) *Short Orders*	7½-oz. can	340
(Libby's):		
Beef	⅓ cup	110
Pork	⅓ cup	120

Food and Description	Measure or Quantity	Calories
Manwich (Hunt's)	1 serving	310
Frozen (Banquet) *Cookin' Bag*	5-oz. pkg.	199
SLOPPY JOE SAUCE		
(Ragú) *Joe Sauce*	3½ oz.	50
SLOPPY JOE SEASONING MIX:		
*(Durkee) pizza flavor	1¼ cups	746
(French's)	1 pkg.	128
*(Hunt's) *Manwich*	5.9-oz. serving	320
SNACK BAR (Pepperidge Farm):		
Apple nut, apricot-raspberry or blueberry	1.7-oz. piece	170
Brownie nut or date nut	1½-oz. piece	190
Chocolate chip or coconut macaroon	1½-oz. piece	210
SOAVE WINE (Antinori)	3 fl. oz.	84
SOFT DRINK:		
Sweetened:		
Apple (Slice)	6 fl. oz.	98
Birch beer (Canada Dry)	6 fl. oz.	82
Bitter lemon:		
(Canada Dry)	6 fl. oz.	75
(Schweppes)	6 fl. oz.	82
Bubble Up	6 fl. oz.	73
Cactus Cooler (Canada Dry)	6 fl. oz.	90
Cherry:		
(Canada Dry) wild	6 fl. oz.	98
(Shasta) black	6 fl. oz.	81
Cherry-lime (Spree)	6 fl. oz.	79
Chocolate (Yoo-Hoo)	6 fl. oz.	93
Citrus mist (Shasta)	6 fl. oz.	85
Club	Any quantity	0
Cola:		
Coca-Cola:		
Regular or caffeine-free	6 fl. oz.	71
Classic	6 fl. oz.	61
Jamaica (Canada Dry)	6 fl. oz.	79
Pepsi-Cola, regular or *Pepsi Free*	6 fl. oz.	80
(Shasta) regular	6 fl. oz.	72
(Slice) cherry	6 fl. oz.	82
(Spree)	6 fl. oz.	73
Collins mix (Canada Dry)	6 fl. oz.	60
Cream:		
(Canada Dry) vanilla	6 fl. oz.	97
(Schweppes)	6 fl. oz.	86
Dr. Nehi (Royal Crown)	6 fl. oz.	82
Dr. Pepper	6 fl. oz.	75
Fruit punch:		
(Nehi)	6 fl. oz.	107

Food and Description	Measure or Quantity	Calories
(Shasta)	6 fl. oz.	87
Ginger ale:		
(Canada Dry) regular	6 fl. oz.	68
(Fanta)	6 fl. oz.	60
(Shasta)	6 fl. oz.	60
(Spree)	6 fl. oz.	60
Ginger beer (Schweppes)	6 fl. oz.	70
Grape:		
(Fanta)	6 fl. oz.	81
(Hi-C)	6 fl. oz.	74
(Nehi)	6 fl. oz.	96
(Schweppes)	6 fl. oz.	95
Grapefruit (Spree)	6 fl. oz.	77
Lemon lime:		
(Minute Maid)	6 fl.oz.	67
(Shasta)	6 fl. oz.	73
(Spree)	6 fl. oz.	77
Lemon-tangerine (Spree)	6 fl. oz.	82
Mello Yello	6 fl. oz.	87
Mountain Dew	6 fl. oz.	89
Mr. PiBB	6 fl. oz.	68
Orange:		
(Canada Dry) *Sunrise*	6 fl. oz.	68
(Hi-C)	6 fl. oz.	74
(Slice)	6 fl. oz.	97
Peach (Nehi)	6 fl. oz.	102
Quinine or tonic water		
(Canada Dry; Schweppes)	6 fl. oz.	68
Red Pop (Shasta)	6 fl. oz.	79
Root beer:		
Barrelhead (Canada Dry)	6 fl. oz.	82
(Dad's)	6 fl. oz.	83
Rooti (Canada Dry)	6 fl. oz.	82
(Shasta) draft	6 fl. oz.	77
(Spree)	6 fl. oz.	77
7-Up	6 fl. oz.	72
Slice	6 fl. oz.	76
Sprite	6 fl. oz.	68
Strawberry (Shasta)	6 fl. oz.	73
Tropical blend (Spree)	6 fl. oz.	73
Upper Ten (Royal Crown)	6 fl. oz.	85
Dietetic:		
Apple (Slice)	6 fl. oz.	10
Birch beer (Shasta)	6 fl. oz.	2
Bubble Up	6 fl. oz.	1
Cherry (Shasta) black	6 fl. oz.	0
Chocolate (Shasta)	6 fl. oz.	0
Coffee (No-Cal)	6 fl. oz.	1
Cola:		
(Canada Dry; Shasta)	6 fl. oz.	0

Food and Description	Measure or Quantity	Calories
Coca-Cola, regular or caffeine free	6 fl. oz.	<1
Diet Rite	6 fl. oz.	<1
Pepsi, diet, light or caffeine free	6 fl. oz.	<1
RC	6 fl. oz.	<1
(Slice)	6 fl. oz.	10
Cream (Shasta)	6 fl. oz.	<1
Dr. Pepper	6 fl. oz.	<2
Fresca	6 fl. oz.	2
Ginger ale:		
(Canada Dry)	6 fl. oz.	1
(Schweppes)	6 fl. oz.	2
Grape (Shasta)	6 fl. oz.	0
Grapefruit (Shasta)	6 fl. oz.	2
Kiwi-passionfruit (Schweppes) mid-calorie royals	6 fl. oz.	35
Lemon-lime (*Diet Rite*)	6 fl.oz.	2
Mr. PiBB	6 fl. oz.	<1
Orange:		
(Canada Dry; No-Cal)	6 fl. oz.	1
(Minute Maid)	6 fl. oz.	3
(Shasta)	6 fl. oz.	<1
Peach, *Diet Rite*, golden	6 fl. oz.	1
Peaches 'n cream (Schweppes) mid-calorie royals	6 fl. oz.	35
Quinine or tonic water (No-Cal)	6 fl. oz.	3
Raspberry, *Diet Rite*, red	6 fl. oz.	2
RC 100 (Royal Crown) caffeine free	6 fl. oz.	<1
Red Pop (Shasta)	6 fl. oz.	0
Root beer:		
Barrelhead (Canada Dry)	6 fl. oz.	1
(Dad's; Ramblin'; Shasta)	6 fl. oz.	<1
7-Up	6 fl. oz.	2
Slice	6 fl. oz.	13
Sprite	6 fl. oz.	1
Strawberry-banana (Schweppes) mid-calorie royals	6 fl. oz.	35
Tab, regular or caffeine free	6 fl. oz.	<1
SOLE, frozen:		
(Frionor) *Norway Gourmet*	4-oz. fillet	60
(Healthy Choice):		
Au gratin	11-oz. meal	270
With lemon butter	8¼-oz. meal	230
(Mrs. Paul's) fillets, breaded & fried	6-oz. serving	280
(Van de Kamp's) batter dipped, french fried	1 piece	140
(Weight Watchers) stuffed	10½-oz. meal	310

Food and Description	Measure or Quantity	Calories
SOUFFLE, frozen (Stouffer's):		
Corn	4-oz. serving	160
Spinach	4-oz. serving	140
SOUP:		
Canned, regular pack:		
*Asparagus (Campbell), condensed, cream of:		
Regular	8-oz. serving	90
Creamy Natural	8-oz. serving	200
Bean:		
(Campbell):		
Chunky, with ham, old fashioned	11-oz. can	290
*Condensed, with bacon	8-oz. serving	150
(Grandma Brown's)	8-oz. serving	182
Bean, black:		
*(Campbell) condensed	8-oz. serving	110
(Crosse & Blackwell)	6½-oz. serving	80
Beef:		
(Campbell):		
Chunky:		
Regular	10¾-oz. can	190
Stroganoff	10¾-oz. can	300
*Condensed:		
Regular	8-oz. serving	80
Broth	8-oz. serving	15
Consommé	8-oz. serving	25
Noodle, home style	8-oz. serving	90
(College Inn) broth	1 cup	18
(Progresso):		
Regular	10½-oz. can	180
Hearty	½ of 19-oz. can	160
Tomato, with rotini	½ of 19-oz. can	170
Vegetable	10½-oz. can	160
(Swanson) broth	7¼-oz. can	20
Beef barley (Progresso)	10½-oz. can	170
Beef cabbage (Manischewitz)	1 cup	62
*Broccoli (Campbell) condensed, *Creamy Natural*	8-oz. serving	140
Celery:		
*(Campbell) condensed, cream of	8-oz. serving	100
*(Rokeach):		
Prepared with milk	10-oz. serving	190
Prepared with water	10-oz. serving	90
*Cheddar cheese (Campbell)	8-oz. serving	130
Chickarina (Progresso)	½ of 19-oz. can	130
Chicken:		
(Campbell):		

176

Food and Description	Measure or Quantity	Calories
Chunky:		
& rice	19-oz. can	280
vegetable	19-oz. can	340
*Condensed:		
Alphabet	8-oz. serving	80
Broth:		
Plain	8-oz. serving	35
& rice	8-oz. serving	50
Cream of	8-oz. serving	110
Gumbo	8-oz. serving	60
Mushroom, creamy	8-oz. serving	120
Noodle:		
Regular	8-oz. serving	70
NoodleOs	8-oz. serving	70
& rice	8-oz. serving	60
Vegetable	8-oz. serving	70
*Semi-condensed, Soup For One,		
Vegetable, full flavored	11-oz. serving	120
(College Inn) broth	1 cup	35
(Hain) broth	8¾-oz. serving	70
(Manischewitz):		
Clear	1 cup	46
Rice	1 cup	83
Vegetable	1 cup	55
(Progresso):		
Broth	4-oz. serving	8
Cream of	½ of 19-oz. can	180
Hearty	10½-oz. can	130
(Swanson) broth	7¼-oz. can	30
Chili beef (Campbell) Chunky	11-oz. can	290
Chowder:		
Beef'n vegetable (Hormel) Short Orders	7½-oz. can	120
Clam:		
Manhattan style:		
(Campbell):		
Chunky	19-oz. can	300
*Condensed	8-oz. serving	70
(Crosse & Blackwell)	6½-oz. serving	50
(Progresso)	½ of 19-oz. can	120
*(Snow's) condensed	7½-oz. serving	70
New England style:		
*(Campbell):		
Condensed:		
Made with milk	8-oz. serving	150
Made with water	8-oz. serving	80
Semi-condensed,		

Food and Description	Measure or Quantity	Calories
Soup For One:		
Made with milk	11-oz. serving	190
Made with water	11-oz. serving	130
(Crosse & Blackwell)	6½-oz. serving	90
*(Gorton's)	1 can	560
(Hain)	9¼-oz. serving	180
(Progresso)	10½-oz. can	240
*(Snow's) condensed, made with milk	7½-oz. serving	140
Corn (Progresso)	½ of 18½-oz. can	200
*Fish (Snow's) condensed, made with milk	7½-oz. serving	130
Ham'n potato (Hormel)	7½-oz. can	130
Consommé madrilene (Crosse & Blackwell)	6½-oz. serving	25
Crab (Crosse & Blackwell)	6½-oz. serving	50
Escarole (Progresso)	½ of 18½-oz. can	30
Gazpacho (Crosse & Blackwell)	6½-oz. serving	30
Ham'n butter bean (Campbell) *Chunky*	10¾-oz. can	·280
Italian vegetable pasta (Hain)	9½-oz. serving	160
Lentil:		
(Hain) vegetarian	9½-oz. serving	160
(Progresso) with sausage	½ of 19-oz. can	180
Macaroni & bean (Progresso)	10½-oz. can	180
*Meatball alphabet (Campbell) condensed	8-oz. serving	100
Minestrone:		
(Campbell):		
Chunky	19-oz. can	280
*Condensed	8-oz. serving	80
(Hain)	9½-oz. serving	170
(Progresso):		
Beef	10½-oz. can	190
Chicken	½ of 19-oz. can	130
Zesty	½ of 19-oz. can	150
Mushroom:		
*(Campbell):		
Condensed:		
Cream of	8-oz. serving	100
Golden	8-oz. serving	80
(Crosse & Blackwell) cream of, bisque	6½-oz. serving	90
*(Rokeach) cream of:		
Prepared with milk	10-oz. serving	240
Prepared with water	10-oz. serving	150
*Noodle (Campbell) & ground beef	8-oz. serving	90
*Onion (Campbell):		
Regular	8-oz. serving	60

Food and Description	Measure or Quantity	Calories
Cream of:		
Made with water	8-oz. serving	100
Made with water & milk	8-oz. serving	140
*Oyster stew (Campbell):		
Made with milk	8-oz. serving	150
Made with water	8-oz. serving	80
*Pea, green (Campbell)	8-oz. serving	160
Pea, split:		
(Campbell):		
Chunky, with ham	19-oz. can	400
*Condensed, with		
ham & bacon	8-oz. serving	160
(Grandma Brown's)	8-oz. serving	184
*Pepper pot (Campbell)	8-oz. serving	90
*Potato (Campbell) cream of:		
Regular:		
Made with water	8-oz. serving	70
Made with water & milk	8-oz. serving	110
Creamy Natural	8-oz. serving	220
Shav (Gold's)	8-oz. serving	25
Shrimp:		
*(Campbell) condensed,		
cream of:		
Made with milk	8-oz. serving	160
Made with water	8-oz. serving	90
(Crosse & Blackwell)	6½-oz. serving	90
*Spinach (Campbell) condensed,		
Creamy Natural	8-oz. serving	160
Steak & potato (Campbell)		
Chunky	19-oz. can	340
Tomato:		
(Campbell):		
Condensed:		
Regular:		
Made with milk	8-oz. serving	160
Made with water	8-oz. serving	90
& rice, old fashioned	8-oz. serving	110
Creamy Natural	8-oz. serving	190
Semi-condensed,		
Soup For One, Royale	11-oz. serving	180
(Manischewitz)	1 cup	60
(Progresso)	½ of 19-oz. can	120
*(Rokeach):		
Made with milk	10-oz. serving	190
Made with water	10-oz. serving	90
Tortellini (Progresso):		
Regular	½ of 19-oz. can	90
Turkey (Campbell) *Chunky*	18¾-oz. can	300

179

Food and Description	Measure or Quantity	Calories
Vegetable:		
(Campbell):		
Chunky:		
Regular	19-oz. can	260
Beef, old fashioned	19-oz. can	320
*Condensed:		
Regular	8-oz. serving	80
Beef or vegetarian	10-oz. serving	70
*Semi-condensed,		
Soup For One, old world	11-oz. serving	160
(Hain):		
Chicken	9½-oz. serving	120
Vegetarian	9½-oz. serving	140
(Manischewitz)	1 cup	63
(Progresso)	½ of 19-oz. can	80
*(Rokeach) vegetarian	10-oz. serving	90
Vichyssoise (Crosse & Blackwell)	6½-oz. serving	70
*Won ton (Campbell)	8-oz. serving	40
Canned, dietetic pack:		
Bean (Pritikin) navy	½ of 14¾-oz. can	130
Beef (Campbell) *Chunky,*		
& mushroom, low sodium	10¾-oz. can	210
Chicken:		
(Campbell) low sodium:		
Regular, with noodles	10¾-oz. can	160
Vegetable	10¾-oz. can	240
*(Estee) & vegetable, chunky	7½-oz. serving	130
(Hain) noodle, no salt added	9½-oz. serving	110
(Pritikin):		
Broth	½ of 13¾-oz. can	14
Vegetable	½ of 14¾-oz. can	70
(Weight Watchers) noodle	10½-oz. can	80
Chowder (Pritikin):		
Manhattan	½ of 14¾-oz. can	70
New England	½ of 14¾-oz. can	118
Lentil (Pritikin)	½ of 14¾-oz. can	100
*Minestrone (Estee)	7½-oz. serving	165
Mushroom (Campbell) cream of,		
low sodium	10½-oz. can	200
Onion (Campbell) low sodium	10½-oz. can	80
Pea, split (Campbell) low sodium	10¾-oz. can	240
Tomato: (Campbell) low sodium		
with tomato pieces	10½-oz. can	180
Turkey:		
(Hain) & rice, no salt added	9½-oz. serving	100
(Pritikin) vegetable	½ of 14¾-oz. can	50
(Weight Watchers) vegetable	10½-oz. can	70
Vegetable:		
(Campbell) *Chunky,* low		

Food and Description	Measure or Quantity	Calories
sodium, vegetarian	10¾-oz. serving	170
(Hain) vegetarian, no salt added	9½-oz. serving	150
(Pritikin)	½ of 14¾-oz. can	70
(Weight Watchers) vegetarian, chunky	10½-oz. can	100
Frozen:		
Asparagus (Kettle Ready) cream of	6 fl. oz.	62
*Barley & mushroom:		
(Empire Kosher)	7½-oz. serving	69
(Tabatchnick)	8-oz. serving	92
Bean (Kettle Ready) black	6 fl. oz.	154
Bean & barley (Tabatchnick)	8 oz.	63
Beef (Kettle Ready) vegetable	6 fl. oz.	85
Broccoli, cream of:		
(Kettle Ready) regular	6 oz.	95
(Tabatchnick)	7½ oz.	90
Cheese, cheddar (Kettle Ready)	6 oz.	158
Chicken:		
(Empire Kosher) noodle	7½-oz. serving	267
(Kettle Ready):		
Cream of	6 fl. oz.	98
Gumbo	6 fl. oz.	93
Chowder:		
Clam:		
Boston (Kettle Ready)	6 oz.	131
Manhattan:		
(Kettle Ready)	6 oz.	69
(Tabatchnick)	7½ oz.	94
New England:		
(Kettle Ready)	6 oz.	116
(Stouffer's)	8 oz.	180
(Tabatchnick)	7½ oz.	97
Corn & broccoli (Kettle Ready)	6 oz.	101
Minestrone (Tabatchnick)	8 oz.	147
Mushroom (Kettle Ready) cream of	6 fl. oz.	85
Onion (Kettle Ready)	6 oz.	42
Pea, split with ham:		
(Kettle Ready)	6 oz.	155
(Tabatchnick)	8 oz.	186
Potato (Kettle Ready) cream of	8 oz.	162
Spinach, cream of:		
(Stouffer's)	8 oz.	210
(Tabatchnick)	7½ oz.	90
Tomato (Empire Kosher) rice, cream of	7½ oz.	227
Vegetable:		
(Empire Kosher)	7½ oz.	111
(Kettle Ready) garden	6 oz.	85

Food and Description	Measure or Quantity	Calories
(Tabatchnick)	8 oz.	97
*Won Ton (La Choy)	½ of 15-oz. pkg.	50
Mix, regular:		
*Asparagus (Knorr)	8 fl. oz.	80
*Barley (Knorr) country	10 fl. oz.	120
Beef:		
*(Lipton) *Cup-A-Soup:*		
Noodle	6 fl. oz.	44
Lots-A-Noodles	7 fl. oz.	111
*Broccoli (Lipton) *Cup-A-Soup,* creamy:		
Regular	6 fl. oz.	62
Cheese	6 fl. oz.	69
*Cauliflower (Knorr)	8 fl. oz.	100
*Cheese & broccoli (Hain)	¾ cup	310
*Chicken:		
*(Knorr) noodle	8 fl. oz.	100
(Lipton):		
Cup-A-Broth	6 fl. oz.	25
Cup-A-Soup, & rice	6 fl. oz.	45
Country style, hearty	6 fl. oz.	73
Lots-A-Noodles, regular	7 fl. oz.	120
*Chowder (Gorton's) New England	¼ of can	140
*Herb (Knorr) fine	8 fl. oz.	130
*Hot & sour (Knorr)	8 fl. oz.	80
*Leek (Knorr)	8 fl. oz.	110
*Lentil (Hain) savory	¾ cup	130
*Minestrone:		
(Hain)	¾ cup	110
(Knorr) hearty	10 fl. oz.	130
(Manischewitz)	6 fl. oz.	50
*Mushroom:		
*(Knorr)	8 fl. oz.	100
(Lipton):		
Regular, beef	8 fl. oz.	40
Cup-A-Soup, cream of	6 fl. oz.	82
*Noodle (Lipton):		
With chicken broth	8 fl. oz.	70
Giggle Noodle	8 fl. oz.	80
*Onion:		
*(Hain)	¾ cup	50
*(Knorr) french	8 fl. oz.	50
(Lipton):		
Regular, beef	8 fl. oz.	35
Cup-A-Soup	6 fl. oz.	30
*Oxtail (Knorr) hearty beef	8 fl. oz.	70
*Pea, green (Lipton) *Cup-A-Soup*	6 fl. oz.	115
*Pea, split (Hain)	¾ cup	310

Food and Description	Measure or Quantity	Calories
*Tomato (Lipton) *Cup-A-Soup*	6 fl. oz.	100
*Tomato onion (Lipton)	8 fl. oz.	80
*Tortellini (Knorr)	8 fl. oz.	60
*Vegetable:		
(Hain)	¾ cup	80
(Knorr) spring, with herbs	8 fl. oz.	30
(Lipton):		
Regular, country	8 fl. oz.	80
Cup-A-Soup:		
Regular, spring	6 fl. oz.	41
Country style, harvest	6 fl. oz.	94
Lots-A-Noodles, garden	7 fl. oz.	130
(Manischewitz)	6 fl. oz.	50
(Southland) frozen	⅕ of 16-oz. pkg.	60
Mix, dietetic:		
Beef:		
*(Estee) noodle	6 fl. oz.	20
(Weight Watchers) broth	1 packet	8
*Broccoli (Lipton) *Cup-A-Soup,* lite, golden	6 fl. oz.	42
Chicken noodle, *(Estee)	6 fl. oz.	25
*Mushroom:		
(Estee) cream of	6 fl. oz.	40
(Hain) no added salt	¾ cup	250
*Onion:		
(Estee)	6 fl. oz.	25
(4C) reduced salt	8 fl. oz.	30
(Hain) no salt added	¾ cup	50
*Tomato (Estee)	6 fl. oz.	40
SOUP GREENS (Durkee)	2⅓-oz. jar	216
SOUTHERN COMFORT:		
80 proof	1 fl. oz.	79
100 proof	1 fl. oz.	95
SOYBEAN CURD OR TOFU	2¾″ × 1½″ × 1″cake	86
SOYBEAN OR NUT:		
Dry roasted (*Soy Ahoy; Soy Town*)	1 oz.	139
Oil roasted (*Soy Ahoy; Soy Town*) plain, barbecue or garlic	1 oz.	152
SPAGHETTI:		
Dry (Pritikin) whole wheat	1 oz.	110
Cooked:		
8-10 minutes, "Al Dente"	1 cup	216
14-20 minutes, tender	1 cup	155
Canned:		
(Franco-American):		
In meat sauce	7½-oz. can	210
With meatballs in tomato sauce, *SpaghettiOs*	7⅜-oz. can	210

Food and Description	Measure or Quantity	Calories
With sliced franks in tomato sauce, *SpaghettiOs* (Hormel) *Short Orders*, &	7⅜-oz. can	210
meatballs in tomato sauce	7½-oz. can	210
(Libby's) & meatballs in tomato sauce	7½-oz. serving	189
Dietetic (Estee) & meatballs	7½-oz. serving	240
Frozen:		
(Armour Classics) *Dining Lite*, with meat	9-oz. meal	220
(Banquet) & meat sauce	8-oz. pkg.	270
(Morton) & meatball	10-oz. dinner	200
(Stouffer's) *Lean Cuisine*	11½-oz. pkg.	280
(Weight Watchers) with meat sauce	10½-oz. meal	280
SPAGHETTI SAUCE, canned:		
Regular pack:		
Alfredo (Progresso), seafood	½ cup	220
Bolognese (Progresso)	½ cup	150
Chunky (Hunt's)	4-oz. serving	50
Clam (Progresso) white, authentic pasta sauce	½ cup	130
Garden Style (Ragú)	4-oz. serving	80
Homestyle (Hunt's)	4 oz.	60
Lobster (Progresso) rock	½ cup	120
Marinara:		
(Prince)	4-oz. serving	80
(Progresso):		
Regular	½ cup	90
Authentic pasta sauce	½ cup	110
(Ragú)	5-oz. serving	120
Meat or meat flavored:		
(Hunt's)	4-oz. serving	70
(Prego)	4-oz. serving	150
(Ragú) regular	4-oz. serving	80
Meatless or plain:		
(Prego)	4-oz. serving	140
(Ragú) regular	4-oz. serving	80
Mushroom:		
(Hain)	4-oz. serving	80
(Hunt's) regular	4-oz. serving	70
(Prego Plus)	4-oz. serving	130
(Progresso)	½ cup	110
(Ragú) Extra Thick & Zesty	4-oz. serving	110
Primavera (Progresso) creamy	½ cup	190
Romano (Progresso) creamy	½ cup	220

Food and Description	Measure or Quantity	Calories
Sausage & green pepper (Prego Plus)	4-oz. serving	170
Seafood (Progresso):		
Regular	½ cup	110
Authentic pasta sauce	½ cup	190
Sicilian (Progresso)	½ cup	30
Traditional (Hunt's)	4 oz.	70
Veal (Prego Plus)	4-oz. serving	150
Dietetic pack:		
(Estee)	4-oz. serving	60
(Furman's) low sodium	½ cup	83
(Prego) low sodium	½ cup	100
(Pritikin) plain or mushroom	4-oz. serving	60
(Weight Watchers) mushroom	⅓ cup	40
SPAGHETTI SAUCE MIX:		
*(Durkee) regular	½ cup	45
*(French's) with mushrooms	⅝ cup	100
(Lawry's) rich & thick	1½-oz. pkg.	147
*(Spatini)	½ cup	84
SPAM, luncheon meat (Hormel):		
Regular, smoke flavored or with cheese chunks	1-oz. serving	85
Deviled	1 T.	35
SPARKLING COOLER CITRUS, La Croix (Heilemann)	6 fl. oz.	107
SPECIAL K, cereal (Kellogg's)	1 cup (1 oz.)	110
SPINACH:		
Fresh, whole leaves	½ cup	4
Boiled	½ cup	18
Canned, regular pack (Allens) solids & liq.	½ cup	25
Canned, dietetic pack (Del Monte) No Salt Added	½ cup	25
Frozen:		
(Birds Eye):		
Chopped or leaf	⅓ pkg.	28
Creamed	⅓ pkg.	60
(Green Giant):		
Creamed	3.3 oz.	40
Harvest Fresh	4.5 oz. serving	25
(McKenzie) chopped or cut	⅓ pkg.	25
SPINACH PUREE, canned (Larsen) low sodium	½ cup	22
SQUASH, SUMMER:		
Fresh, yellow, boiled slices	½ cup	13
Fresh, zucchini, boiled slices	½ cup	9
Canned (Progresso) zucchini, in tomato sauce	½ cup	50

185

Food and Description	Measure or Quantity	Calories
Frozen:		
(Birds Eye) zucchini	⅓ pkg.	19
(Larsen) yellow crookneck	3.3 oz.	18
(McKenzie) crookneck	⅓ pkg.	20
(Mrs. Paul's) sticks,		
batter dipped, french fried	⅓ pkg.	180
(Ore-Ida) breaded	3 oz.	150
SQUASH, WINTER:		
Acorn, baked	½ cup	56
Hubbard, baked, mashed	½ cup	51
Frozen:		
(Birds Eye)	⅓ pkg.	43
(Southland) butternut	4-oz. serving	45
STEAK (See BEEF)		
STEAK & GREEN PEPPERS,		
frozen:		
(Green Giant)	9-oz. entree	250
(Swanson)	8½-oz. entree	200
STEAK UMM	2 oz.	180
STOCK BASE (French's) beef		
or chicken	1 tsp.	8
STRAWBERRY:		
Fresh, capped	½ cup	26
Frozen (Birds Eye):		
Halves	⅓ pkg.	164
Whole	¼ pkg.	89
Whole, quick thaw	½ pkg.	125
STRAWBERRY FRUIT JUICE,		
canned (Smucker's)	8 fl. oz.	120
STRAWBERRY NECTAR, canned		
(Libby's)	6 fl. oz.	60
STRAWBERRY PRESERVE		
OR JAM:		
Sweetened:		
(Bama)	1 T.	45
(Smucker's)	1 T.	53
(Welch's)	1 T.	52
Dietetic or low calorie:		
(Estee; Louis Sherry)	1 T.	6
(Diet Delight)	1 T.	12
(Featherweight) calorie reduced	1 T.	16
STUFFING MIX:		
*Beef, *Stove Top*	½ cup	180
*Chicken:		
*(Bell's)	½ cup	224
*(Betty Crocker)	⅕ pkg.	180
Stove Top	½ cup	180
*Cornbread, *Stove Top*	½ cup	170

Food and Description	Measure or Quantity	Calories
Cube or herb seasoned (Pepperidge Farm)	1 oz.	110
*Herb (Betty Crocker) traditional	⅙ pkg.	190
*Pork, *Stove Top*	½ cup	170
*Premium Blend (Bell's)	½ cup	180
*Ready Mix (Bell's)	½ cup	224
White bread (Mrs. Cubbison's)	1 oz.	101
STURGEON, smoked	4-oz. serving	169
SUCCOTASH:		
Canned:		
(Comstock) whole kernel	½ cup	80
(Larsen) *Freshlike*	½ cup	80
(Libby's) cream style	½ cup	111
(Stokely-Van Camp)	½ cup	85
Frozen:		
(Birds Eye)	⅓ pkg.	104
(Frosty Acres)	3.3 oz.	100
***SUDDENLY SALADS** (General Mills):*		
Macaroni, creamy	⅙ pkg.	200
Pasta, Italian	⅙ pkg.	160
Potato, creamy	⅙ pkg.	250
SUGAR:		
Brown, dark or light	1 T.	48
Confectioners	1 T.	30
Granulated	1 T.	46
Maple	1¾″ × 1¼″ × ½″ piece	104
SUGAR SUBSTITUTE:		
(Estee)	1 tsp.	12
(Featherweight)	3 drops	0
(Pritikin) *Supreme*	1.76-oz. packet	3
Sprinkle Sweet (Pillsbury)	1 tsp.	2
Sweet'n-it (Estee) liquid	5 drops	0
Sweet 'N Low:		
Brown	1 tsp.	20
Granulated	1-gram packet	4
Liquid	1 drop	0
***SUGAR PUFFS,** cereal* (Malt-O-Meal)	⅞ cup	110
***SUKIYAKI DINNER** (Chun King) stir fry*	6 oz.	257
SUNFLOWER SEED (Fisher):		
In hull, roasted, salted	1 oz.	86
Hulled, dry roasted, salted	1 oz.	164
Hulled, oil roasted, salted	1 oz.	167
***SUNTOPS** (Dole)*	1 bar	40

187

Food and Description	Measure or Quantity	Calories
SURIMI (See CRAB SUBSTITUTE)		
SWEETBREADS, calf, braised	4-oz. serving	191
SWEET POTATO:		
Baked, peeled	5″ × 1″ potato	155
Canned:		
(Allen's)	4-oz. serving	50
(Joan of Arc):		
Mashed	½ cup	90
Whole:		
Candied	½ cup	240
Heavy syrup	½ cup	130
In pineapple-orange sauce	½ cup	210
(Trappey's) *Sugary Sam:*		
Cut	½ cup (4.3 oz.)	110
Whole	½ cup (4.3 oz.)	130
Frozen:		
(Mrs. Paul's) candied, with apples	4-oz. serving	150
(Stouffer's) & apples	5-oz. serving	160
SWEET 'N SOUR COCKTAIL MIX		
(Holland House) liquid	1 fl. oz.	34
SWEET & SOUR PORK, frozen:		
(Chun King)	13-oz. entree	400
(La Choy)	12-oz. entree	360
SWISS STEAK, frozen (Swanson)	10-oz. dinner	350
SWORDFISH, broiled	3″ × 3″ × ½″ steak	218
SYRUP (See also TOPPING):		
Regular:		
Blackberry (Smucker's)	1 T.	50
Boysenberry (Smucker's)	1 T.	50
Chocolate or chocolate-flavored:		
Bosco	1 T.	55
(Hershey's)	1 T.	40
(Nestlé) *Quik*	1 oz.	80
Corn, *Karo,* dark or light	1 T.	60
Maple, *Karo,* imitation	1 T.	57
Pancake or waffle:		
(Aunt Jemima)	1 T.	53
Golden Griddle	1 T.	54
Karo	1 T.	58
Log Cabin, regular or buttered	1 T.	72
Mrs. Butterworth's	1 T.	55
(Smucker's)	1-oz. packet	116
Strawberry (Smucker's)	1 T.	50
Dietetic or low calorie:		
Blueberry (Estee)	1 T.	8
Chocolate or chocolate-flavored (Estee)	1 T.	20
Maple (S&W) *Nutradiet*	1 T.	12

Food and Description	Measure or Quantity	Calories
Pancake or waffle:		
(Aunt Jemima)	1 T.	29
(Cary's)	1 T.	6
(Estee)	1 T.	8
Log Cabin	1 T.	34
(Weight Watchers)	1 T.	25

T

Food and Description	Measure or Quantity	Calories
TACO:		
*(Ortega)	1 oz.	54
*Mix (Durkee)	½ cup	321
Shell (Ortega)	1 shell	50
TACO BELL RESTAURANTS:		
Burrito:		
Bean:		
Green sauce	6¾-oz. serving	351
Red sauce	6¾-oz. serving	357
Beef:		
Green sauce	6¾-oz. serving	398
Red sauce	6¾-oz. serving	403
Supreme:		
Regular:		
Green sauce	8½-oz. serving	407
Red sauce	8½-oz. serving	413
Double beef:		
Green sauce	9-oz. serving	451
Red sauce	9-oz. serving	456
Cinnamon crispas	1.7-oz. serving	259
Enchirito:		
Green sauce	7½-oz. serving	371
Red sauce	7½-oz. serving	382
Fajita:		
Chicken	4¾-oz. serving	225
Steak	4¾-oz. serving	234
Guacamole	¾-oz. serving	34
Meximelt	3¾-oz. serving	266
Nachos:		
Regular	3¾-oz. serving	345
Bellgrande	10.1-oz. serving	648
Pepper, jalapeno	3½-oz. serving	20
Pico De Gallo	1-oz. serving	8
Pintos & cheese:		
Green sauce	4½-oz. serving	184
Red sauce	4½-oz. serving	190
Pizza, Mexican	7.9-oz. serving	575
Ranch dressing	2.6-oz. serving	235

Food and Description	Measure or Quantity	Calories
Salsa	.3-oz. serving	18
Sour cream	¾-oz. serving	46
Taco:		
Regular	2¾-oz. serving	183
Bellgrande	5¾-oz. serving	355
Light	6-oz. serving	410
Soft:		
Regular	3¼-oz. serving	338
Supreme	4.4-oz. serving	275
Super combo	5-oz. serving	286
Taco salad:		
With shell	18.7-oz. serving	502
With salsa:		
Regular	21-oz. serving	941
Without shell	18.7-oz. serving	520
Taco sauce:		
Regular	.4-oz. packet	2
Hot	.4-oz. packet	2
Tostada:		
Green sauce	5½-oz. serving	237
Red sauce	5½-oz. serving	243
TACO JOHN'S RESTAURANTS:		
Burrito:		
Bean	5-oz. serving	197
Beef	5-oz. serving	303
Chicken:		
Regular	5-oz. serving	227
With green chili	12¼-oz. serving	344
Combo	5-oz. serving	250
Smothered:		
With green chili	12¼-oz. serving	367
With Texas chili	12¼-oz. serving	455
Super:		
Regular	8¼-oz. serving	389
With chicken	8¼-oz. serving	366
Chimichanga:		
Regular	12-oz. serving	464
With chicken	12-oz. serving	441
Mexican rice	8-oz. serving	340
Nachos:		
Regular	5-oz. serving	468
Super	11¼-oz. serving	669
Potato Ole, large	6-oz. serving	414
Taco:		
Regular	4¼-oz. serving	178
With chicken	4¼-oz. serving	140
Softshell:		
Regular	5-oz. serving	224
With chicken	5-oz. serving	180

Food and Description	Measure or Quantity	Calories
Taco Bravo:		
Regular	6¾-oz. serving	319
Super	8-oz. serving	361
Taco burger	6-oz. serving	281
Taco salad:		
Regular:		
Without dressing	6-oz. serving	229
With dressing	8-oz. serving	359
Chicken:		
Without dressing	12¼-oz. serving	377
With dressing	14¼-oz. serving	507
Super:		
Without dressing	12¼-oz. serving	428
With dressing	14¼-oz. serving	558
TAMALE:		
Canned:		
(Hormel) beef, *Short Orders*	7½-oz. can	270
(Old El Paso)	1 tamale	95
(Pride of Mexico) beef	1 tamale	115
Frozen (Hormel) beef	1 tamale	130
TANG:		
Canned, *Fruit Box:*		
Cherry or strawberry	8.45-fl.-oz. container	121
Grape	8.45-fl.-oz. container	131
Mixed fruit	8.45-fl.-oz. container	137
Orange, regular	8.45-fl.-oz. container	127
*Mix:		
Regular	6 fl. oz.	86
Dietetic	6 fl. oz.	5
TANGERINE OR MANDARIN ORANGE:		
Fresh (Sunkist)	1 large tangerine	39
Canned, solids & liq.:		
Regular pack (Dole)	½ cup	70
Dietetic pack:		
(Diet Delight) juice pack	½ cup	50
(Featherweight) water pack	½ cup	35
(S&W) *Nutradiet*	½ cup	28
TANGERINE DRINK, canned (Hi-C)	6 fl. oz.	90
TANGERINE JUICE, frozen (Minute Maid)	6 fl. oz.	91
TAPIOCA, dry, *Minute,* quick cooking	1 T.	32
TAQUITO, frozen (Van de Kamp's) beef	8-oz. serving	490
TARRAGON (French's)	1 tsp.	5
TASTEEOS, cereal (Ralston Purina)	1¼ cups (1 oz.)	110

Food and Description	Measure or Quantity	Calories
*TEA:		
Bag:		
(Celestial Seasonings):		
After dinner:		
Amaretto Nights or *Swiss Mint*	1 cup	<3
Bavarian Chocolate Orange	1 cup	7
Caffeine free	1 cup	4
Fruit & tea	1 cup	<3
Herb:		
Almond Sunset, Cinnamon apple or *Cranberry Cove*	1 cup	3
Emperor's Choice or *Lemon Zinger*	1 cup	4
Mandarin Orange Spice or *Orange Zinger*	1 cup	5
Roastaroma	1 cup	11
Premium black tea	1 cup	3
(Lipton):		
Plain or flavored	1 cup	2
Herbal:		
Almond pleasure or cinnamon apple	1 cup	2
Quietly chamomile or toasty spice	1 cup	6
(Sahadi) spearmint	1 cup	4
Instant (Nestea)100%	6 fl. oz.	0
TEA MIX, ICED:		
*(4C)	8 fl. oz.	90
*(Lipton) lemon & sugar flavored	1 cup	60
*Nestea, lemon-flavored	1 cup	6
*Dietetic, *Crystal Light*	8 fl. oz.	3
TEQUILA SUNRISE COCKTAIL,		
(Mr. Boston) 12½% alcohol	3 fl. oz.	120
TERIYAKI:		
*Canned (La Choy) chicken	¾ cup	85
Frozen:		
(Chun King)	13-oz. entree	380
(La Choy) Fresh & Light	10-oz. meal	240
(Stouffer's) beef	9¾-oz. serving	290
TERIYAKI BASTE & GLAZE		
(Kikkoman)	1 T.	24
*TEXTURED VEGETABLE PROTEIN,		
Morningstar Farms:		
Breakfast link	1 link	73
Breakfast patties	1 patty	100
Breakfast strips	1 strip	37
Grillers	1 patty	190

Food and Description	Measure or Quantity	Calories
THURINGER:		
(Eckrich) *Smoky Tang*	1-oz. serving	80
(Hormel):		
Beefy	1-oz. serving	100
Old Smokehouse	1-oz. serving	100
(Louis Rich) turkey	1-oz. serving	50
(Ohse) beef	1 oz.	80
(Oscar Mayer) beef	.8-oz. slice	69
TOASTER CAKE OR PASTRY:		
Pop-Tarts (Kellogg's):		
Regular:		
Blueberry, brown sugar, cinnamon or cherry	1 pastry	210
Strawberry	1 pastry	200
Frosted:		
Blueberry, chocolate fudge or strawberry	1 pastry	200
Brown sugar cinnamon, cherry	1 pastry	210
Toaster Strudel (Pillsbury)	1 slice	190
Toastettes (Nabisco) regular or frosted	1 piece	200
Toast-R-Cake (Thomas'):		
Blueberry	1 piece	108
Bran	1 piece	103
Corn	1 piece	120
TOASTY O'S, cereal (Malt-O-Meal)	1¼ cup	107
TOFUTTI:		
Frozen:		
Regular:		
Chocolate supreme or wildberry supreme	4 fl. oz.	210
Maple walnut	4 fl. oz.	230
Vanilla	4 fl. oz.	200
Cuties:		
Chocolate	1 piece	140
Vanilla	1 piece	130
Lite Lite	4 fl. oz.	90
Love Drops:		
Cappuccino or chocolate	4 fl. oz.	230
Vanilla	4 fl. oz.	220
Soft serve:		
Regular	4 fl. oz.	158
Hi-Lite:		
Chocolate	4 fl. oz.	100
Vanilla	4 fl. oz.	90
TOMATO:		
Regular, whole	1 med. tomato	33
Cherry, whole	4 pieces	14

Food and Description	Measure or Quantity	Calories
Canned, regular pack, solids & liq.:		
Angela Mia (Hunt's) crushed	4 oz.	35
(Contadina) sliced, baby	½ cup	50
(Del Monte) stewed	4 oz.	37
(Hunt's):		
Crushed, Italian	½ cup	40
Pear shaped, Italian	4 oz.	20
Stewed, regular	½ cup (4 oz.)	35
Whole, regular	4 oz.	20
(La Victoria) green, whole	1 oz.	8
Canned, dietetic pack, solids & liq.:		
(Del Monte) No Salt Added	½ cup	35
(Featherweight)	½ cup	20
(Furman's) low sodium	½ cup	72
(Hunt's) whole	4 oz.	20
TOMATO & PEPPER, HOT CHILI,		
(Old El Paso) Jalapeño	¼ cup	13
TOMATO JUICE, canned:		
Regular pack:		
(Ardmore Farms)	6-fl.-oz. can	36
(Campbell; Libby's)	6-fl.-oz. can	35
(Hunt's)	6 fl. oz.	30
Dietetic pack (Diet Delight;		
Featherweight)	6 fl. oz.	35
TOMATO JUICE COCKTAIL,		
canned:		
(Ocean Spray) *Firehouse Jubilee*	6 fl. oz.	44
SnapE-Tom	6 fl. oz.	40
TOMATO PASTE, canned:		
Regular pack:		
(Contadina) Italian	6-oz. serving	210
(Hunt's) Italian style	6 oz.	150
Dietetic (Hunt's) low sodium	6-oz. can	135
TOMATO, PICKLED (Claussen)		
green	1 piece	6
TOMATO PUREE, canned:		
Regular (Contadina) heavy	1 cup	100
Dietetic (Featherweight)	1 cup	90
TOMATO SAUCE, canned:		
(Del Monte):		
Regular or No Salt Added	1 cup	70
Hot	½ cup	40
With tomato bits	1 cup	92
(Furman's)	½ cup	58
(Hunt's):		
Regular or with bits	4 oz.	30
With garlic	4 oz.	70
TOM COLLINS (Mr. Boston)		
12½% alcohol	3 fl. oz.	111

Food and Description	Measure or Quantity	Calories
*TOM COLLINS MIX,		
(Bar-Tender's)	6 fl. oz.	177
TONGUE, beef, braised	4-oz. serving	277
TOPPING:		
Regular:		
Butterscotch (Smucker's)	1 T.	70
Caramel (Smucker's) regular	1 T.	70
Chocolate fudge (Hershey's)	1 T.	50
Fudge, hot (Smucker's)		
special recipe	1 T.	75
Marshmallow (Smucker's)	1 T.	60
Pecans in syrup (Smucker's)	1 T.	65
Pineapple (Smucker's)	1 T.	65
Strawberry (Smucker's)	1 T.	60
Walnuts in syrup (Smucker's)	1 T.	65
Dietetic, chocolate (Smucker's)	1 T.	35
TOPPING, WHIPPED:		
Regular:		
Cool Whip (Birds Eye) dairy	1 T.	16
(Johanna) aerosol	1 T.	8
Lucky Whip, aerosol	1 T.	12
Dietetic (Featherweight)	1 T.	3
*Mix:		
Regular, *Dream Whip*	1 T.	5
Dietetic (D-Zerta; Estee)	1 T.	4
TOP RAMEN, beef (Nissin Foods)	3-oz. serving	390
TORTELLINI, frozen:		
(Buitoni):		
Cheese filled, verdi	2.6-oz. serving	220
Meat filled	2.5-oz. entree	223
(Green Giant) cheese marinara,		
one serving	5½-oz. pkg.	260
(Stouffer's):		
Cheese filled, with tomato sauce	9⅝-oz. meal	360
Veal stuffed, in Alfredo sauce	8⅝-oz. meal	500
TORTILLA (Amigos)	6″ × ⅛″ tortilla	111
TOSTADA, frozen (Van de Kamp's)	8½-oz. serving	530
TOSTADA SHELL (Old El Paso)	1 shell	55
TOTAL, cereal (General Mills)	1 cup (1 oz.)	110
TRIPE, canned (Libby's)	6-oz. serving	290
TRIPLE SEC LIQUEUR		
(Mr. Boston)	1 fl. oz.	79
TRIX, cereal (General Mills)	1 cup	110
TROPICAL CITRUS DRINK,		
chilled or *frozen (Five Alive)	6 fl. oz.	85
*TROPICAL QUENCHER DRINK,		
mix, dietetic, *Crystal Light*	8 fl. oz.	3
TUNA:		
Canned in oil:		

196

Food and Description	Measure or Quantity	Calories
(Bumble Bee):		
Chunk, light, solids & liq.	½ cup	265
Solid, white, solids & liq.	½ cup	285
(Carnation) solids & liq.	6½-oz. can	427
(Progresso) light, solid	⅓ cup	150
Canned in water:		
(Breast O'Chicken)	6½-oz. can	211
(Bumble Bee):		
Chunk, light, solids & liq.	½ cup	117
Solid, white, solids & liq.	½ cup	126
(Featherweight) light, chunk	6½-oz. can	210
*TUNA HELPER (General Mills):		
Au gratin	⅕ pkg.	280
Cold salad	⅕ pkg.	440
Buttery rice	⅕ pkg.	280
Creamy mushroom	⅕ pkg.	220
Creamy noodle or fettucini alfredo	⅕ pkg.	300
Tuna pot pie	⅙ pkg.	420
Tuna tetrazzini	⅕ pkg.	240
TUNA NOODLE CASSEROLE,		
frozen (Stouffer's)	10-oz. meal	310
TUNA PIE, frozen (Banquet)	8-oz. pie	395
TUNA SALAD:		
Home recipe	4-oz. serving	193
Canned (Carnation)	¼ of 7½-oz. can	100
TURF & SURF DINNER, frozen		
(Armour) Classic Lights	10-oz. meal	250
TURKEY:		
Fresh, roasted:		
Flesh & skin	4-oz. serving	253
Dark meat	2½" × 1⅝" × ¼" slice	43
Light meat	4" × 2" × ¼" slice	75
Barbecued (Louis Rich) breast, half	1 oz.	40
Packaged:		
(Carl Buddig):		
Regular	1 oz.	50
Ham or salami	1 oz.	40
Hebrew National, breast	1 oz.	37
(Hormel) breast	1 slice	30
(Louis Rich):		
Turkey bologna	1-oz. slice	60
Turkey cotto salami	1-oz. slice	50
Turkey ham, chopped	1-oz. slice	45
Turkey pastrami	1-oz. slice	35
(Ohse):		
Oven cooked	1 oz.	30
Turkey bologna	1 oz.	70
Turkey salami	1 oz.	50

Food and Description	Measure or Quantity	Calories
(Oscar Mayer) breast oven roasted	.7-oz. slice	23
Smoked (Louis Rich):		
Drumsticks	1 oz. (without bone)	40
Wing drumettes	1 oz. (without bone)	45
TURKEY DINNER OR ENTREE, frozen:		
(Armour) *Dinner Classics*	11½-oz. meal	320
(Banquet)	10½-oz. dinner	390
(Healthy Choice) breast	10½-oz. meal	290
(Morton)	10-oz. dinner	226
(Stouffer's):		
Regular, tetrazzini	10-oz. meal	380
Lean Cuisine, Dijon	9½-oz. meal	270
Right Course, sliced, in curry sauce with rice pilaf	8¾-oz. meal	320
(Swanson):		
Regular	8¾-oz. entree	250
Hungry Man	18½-oz. dinner	590
(Weight Watchers) stuffed, breast	8½-oz. meal	260
TURKEY NUGGET, frozen (Empire Kosher)	¼ of 12-oz. pkg.	255
TURKEY PATTY, frozen (Empire Kosher)	¼ of 12-oz. pkg.	188
TURKEY PIE, frozen:		
(Banquet)	7-oz. pie	510
(Empire Kosher)	8-oz. pie	491
(Morton)	7-oz. pie	420
(Stouffer's)	10-oz. pie	540
(Swanson) chunky	10-oz. pie	530
TURKEY TETRAZZINI, frozen:		
(Stouffer's)	6-oz. serving	240
(Weight Watchers)	10-oz. pkg.	310
TURNIP GREENS, canned		
(Allen's) chopped, solids & liq.	½ cup	20
TURNIP ROOTS, frozen		
(McKenzie) diced	1 oz.	4
TURNOVER:		
Frozen (Pepperidge Farm):		
Apple or cherry	1 turnover	310
Blueberry, peach or raspberry	1 turnover	320
Refrigerated (Pillsbury)	1 turnover	170

U

Food and Description	Measure or Quantity	Calories
ULTRA DIET QUICK (TKI Foods):		
Bar	1.2-oz. bar	130
*Mix:		
Dutch chocolate made with lowfat milk	8 fl. oz.	200
Strawberry delight or vanettor creme	8 fl. oz.	100

V

| --- | --- | --- |
VALPOLICELLA WINE (Antinori)	3 fl. oz.	84
VANDERMINT, liqueur	1 fl. oz.	90
VANILLA EXTRACT		
(Virginia Dare)	1 tsp.	10
VEAL, broiled, medium cooked:		
Loin chop	4 oz.	265
Rib, roasted	4 oz.	305
Steak or cutlet, lean & fat	4 oz.	245
VEAL DINNER, frozen:		
(Armour) *Dinner Classics,*		
parmigiana	11¼-oz. meal	400
(Morton) parmigiana	10-oz. dinner	260
(Swanson) parmigiana,		
Hungry Man	20-oz. dinner	640
(Weight Watchers) parmigiana,		
patty	8.4-oz. meal	220
VEAL STEAK, frozen (Hormel):		
Regular	4-oz. serving	130
Breaded	4-oz. serving	240
VEGETABLE BOUILLON		
(Herb-Ox):		
Cube	1 cube	6
Packet	1 packet	12
VEGETABLE JUICE COCKTAIL:		
Regular:		
(Mott's)	6 fl. oz.	30
(Smucker's)	8 fl. oz.	58
V-8	6 fl. oz.	35
Dietetic:		
(S&W) *Nutradiet,* low sodium	6 fl. oz.	35
V-8, low sodium	6 fl. oz.	40
VEGETABLES, MIXED:		
Canned, regular pack:		
(Del Monte) solids & liq.	½ cup	40

Food and Description	Measure or Quantity	Calories
(La Choy) drained:		
Chinese	⅓ of 14-oz. pkg.	12
Chop Suey	½ cup	9
(Veg-All)	½ cup	35
Canned, dietetic pack:		
(Featherweight)	½ cup	40
(Larsen) *Fresh-Lite*	½ cup	35
Frozen:		
(Birds Eye):		
Regular:		
Broccoli, cauliflower & carrots in cheese sauce	5 oz.	100
Carrots, peas & onions, deluxe	⅓ pkg.	52
Medley, in butter sauce	⅓ of 10-oz. pkg.	62
Farm Fresh:		
Broccoli, cauliflower & carrot strips	3.2 oz.	25
Brussels sprouts, cauliflower & carrots	3.2 oz.	30
Stir Fry, Chinese style	⅓ pkg.	35
(Chun King) chow mein, drained	4 oz.	32
(Frosty Acres):		
Regular	3.3 oz.	65
Dutch	3.2 oz.	30
Oriental	3.2 oz.	25
Soup mix	3 oz.	45
Stew	3 oz.	42
Swiss mix	3 oz.	25
(Green Giant):		
Regular:		
Broccoli, cauliflower & carrots in cheese sauce	½ cup	60
Corn, broccoli bounty	½ cup	60
Harvest Fresh	½ cup	60
Harvest Get Togethers:		
Broccoli-cauliflower medley	½ cup	60
Broccoli fanfare	½ cup	80
(La Choy) stir fry	4 oz.	40
(Larsen):		
Regular or chuckwagon blend	3.3 oz.	70
California blend or Italian blend	3.3 oz.	30
Oriental blend	3.3 oz.	25
(Ore-Ida):		
Medley, breaded	3 oz.	160
Stew vegetables	3 oz.	60
(Southland):		
Gumbo	⅕ of 16-oz. pkg.	40
Stew	4 oz.	60

Food and Description	Measure or Quantity	Calories
VEGETABLE STEW, canned *Dinty Moore* (Hormel)	7½-oz. serving	170
"VEGETARIAN FOODS":		
Canned or dry:		
Chicken, fried (Loma Linda) with gravy	1½-oz. piece	70
Chili (Worthington)	½ cup	177
Choplet (Worthington)	1 choplet	50
Dinner cuts (Loma Linda) drained	1 piece	60
Dinner loaf (Loma Linda)	¼ cup	50
Franks, big (Loma Linda)	1.9-oz. frank	100
Franks, sizzle (Loma Linda)	2.2-oz. frank	85
FriChik (Worthington)	1 piece	75
Little links (Loma Linda) drained	.8-oz. link	40
Non-meatballs (Worthington)	1 meatball	32
Nuteena (Loma Linda)	½″ slice	160
Patty mix (Loma Linda)	¼ cup	50
Prime Stakes	1 slice	171
Proteena (Loma Linda)	½″ slice	140
Sandwich spread (Loma Linda)	1 T.	23
*Soyagen, all purpose powder (Loma Linda)	1 cup	130
Soyameat (Worthington):		
Beef, sliced	1 slice	44
Chicken, diced	1 oz.	40
Soyameal, any kind (Worthington)	1 oz.	120
Stew pack (Loma Linda) drained	2 oz.	70
Super links (Worthington)	1 link	110
Swiss steak with gravy (Loma Linda)	1 steak	140
Vegelona (Loma Linda)	½″ slice	100
Vega-links (Worthington)	1 link	55
Wheat protein	4 oz.	124
Worthington 209	1 slice	58
Frozen:		
Beef pie (Worthington)	1 pie	278
Bologna (Loma Linda)	1 oz.	75
Chicken, fried (Loma Linda)	2-oz. serving	180
Chic-Ketts (Worthington)	1 oz.	53
Corned beef, sliced (Worthington)	1 slice	32
Fri Pats (Worthington)	1 patty	204
Meatballs (Loma Linda)	1 meatball	63
Meatless salami (Worthington)	1 slice	44
Prosage (Worthington)	1 link	60

Food and Description	Measure or Quantity	Calories
Smoked beef, slices (Worthington)	1 slice	14
Wham, roll (Worthington)	1 slice	36
VERMOUTH:		
Dry & extra dry (Lejon; Noilly Pratt)	1 fl. oz.	33
Sweet (Lejon; Taylor)	1 fl. oz.	45
VICHY WATER (Schweppes)	Any quantity	0
VINEGAR, DISTILLED OR CIDER	1 T.	2
VODKA (See DISTILLED LIQUOR)		

W

Food and Description	Measure or Quantity	Calories
WAFFLE, frozen: (See also **PANCAKE & WAFFLE MIX**):		
(Aunt Jemima) jumbo	1 waffle	86
(Eggo):		
Regular:		
Apple cinnamon, blueberry or strawberry	1 waffle	130
Buttermilk or homestyle	1 waffle	120
Common Sense, oat bran, plain	1 waffle	110
Nutri-Grain	1 waffle	130
WALNUT, English or Persian (Diamond A)	1 cup	679
WALNUT FLAVORING, black, imitation (Durkee)	1 tsp.	4
WATER CHESTNUT, canned:		
(Chun King) whole, drained	½ of 8½-oz. can	85
(La Choy) drained	¼ cup	16
WATERCRESS, trimmed	½ cup	3
WATERMELON:		
Wedge	4″ × 8″ wedge	111
Diced	½ cup	21
WELSH RAREBIT:		
Home recipe	1 cup	415
Frozen:		
(Green Giant)	5-oz. serving	219
(Stouffer's)	5-oz. serving	350
WENDY'S RESTAURANTS:		
Bacon, breakfast	1 strip	55
Bacon cheeseburger on white bun	1 serving	460
Breakfast sandwich	1 sandwich	370
Buns:		
Wheat, multi-grain	1 bun	135
White	1 bun	160
Chicken sandwich on multi-grain bun	1 sandwich	320

Food and Description	Measure or Quantity	Calories
Chili:		
Regular	8 oz.	260
Large	12 oz.	390
Condiments:		
Bacon	½ strip	30
Cheese, American	1 slice	70
Onion rings	.3-oz. piece	4
Pickle, dill	4 slices	1
Relish	.3-oz. serving	14
Tomato	1 slice	2
Danish	1 piece	360
Drinks:		
Coffee	6 fl. oz.	2
Cola:		
Regular	12 fl. oz	110
Dietetic	12 fl. oz.	Tr.
Fruit flavored drink	12 fl. oz.	110
Hot chocolate	6 fl. oz.	100
Milk:		
Regular	8 fl. oz.	150
Chocolate	8 fl. oz.	210
Non-cola	12 fl. oz.	100
Orange juice	6 fl. oz.	80
Egg, scrambled	1 order	190
Frosty dairy dessert:		
Small	12 fl. oz.	400
Medium	16 fl. oz.	533
Large	20 fl. oz.	667
Hamburger:		
Double, on white bun	1 serving	560
Kids Meal	1 serving	220
Single:		
On wheat bun	1 serving	340
On white bun	1 serving	350
Omelet:		
Ham & cheese	1 omelet	250
Ham, cheese & mushroom	1 omelet	290
Mushroom, onion & green pepper	1 omelet	210
Potato:		
Baked, hot stuffed:		
Plain	1 potato	250
Broccoli & cheese	1 potato	500
Cheese	1 potato	590
Chicken à la King	1 potato	350
Sour cream & chives	1 potato	460
Stroganoff & sour cream	1 potato	490
French fries	regular order	280
Home fries	1 order	360

Food and Description	Measure or Quantity	Calories
Salad Bar, *Garden Spot:*		
Alfalfa sprouts	2 oz.	20
Bacon bits	⅛ oz.	10
Blueberries, fresh	1 T.	8
Breadstick	1 piece	20
Broccoli	½ cup	14
Cantaloupe	1 piece (2 oz.)	4
Carrot	¼ cup	12
Cauliflower	½ cup	14
Cheese:		
American, imitation	1 oz.	70
Cheddar, imitation	1 oz.	90
Cottage	½ cup	110
Mozzarella, imitation	1 oz.	90
Swiss, imitation	1 oz.	80
Chow mein noodles	¼ cup	60
Coleslaw	½ cup	90
Crouton	1 piece	2
Cucumber	¼ cup	4
Mushroom	¼ cup	6
Onions, red	1 T.	4
Orange, fresh	1 piece	5
Pasta salad	½ cup	134
Peas, green	½ cup	60
Peaches, in syrup	1 piece	8
Peppers:		
Banana or mild pepperoncini	1 T.	18
Bell	¼ cup	4
Jalapeño	1 T.	9
Pineapple chunks in juice	½ cup	80
Tomato	1 oz.	6
Turkey ham	¼ cup	46
Watermelon, fresh	1 piece (1 oz.)	1
Salad dressing:		
Regular:		
Blue cheese	1 T.	60
French, red	1 T.	70
Italian, golden	1 T.	45
Oil	1 T.	130
Ranch	1 T.	80
Thousand Island	1 T.	70
Dietetic:		
Bacon & tomato	1 T.	45
Cucumber, creamy	1 T.	50
Italian	1 T.	25
Thousand Island	1 T.	45
Wine vinegar	1 T.	2
Salad, Side, pick-up window	1 salad	110
Salad, taco	1 salad	390

Food and Description	Measure or Quantity	Calories
Sausage	1 patty	200
Toast:		
Regular, with margarine	1 slice	125
French	1 slice	200
WESTERN DINNER, frozen:		
(Banquet)	11-oz. dinner	630
(Morton) regular	10-oz. dinner	290
(Swanson) *Hungry Man*	17½-oz. dinner	750
WHEAT GERM CEREAL		
(Kretschmer)	¼ cup (1 oz.)	110
WHEAT GERM, RAW (Elam's)	1 T.	28
WHEAT HEARTS, cereal		
(General Mills)	1 oz. (3½ T.)	110
WHEATIES, cereal	1 cup (1 oz.)	100
WHISKEY SOUR COCKTAIL		
(Mr. Boston)	3 fl. oz.	120
***WHISKEY SOUR MIX**		
(Bar-Tender's)	3½ fl. oz.	177
WHITE CASTLE:		
Bun only	.9-oz. bun	74
Cheese only	1 piece	31
Cheeseburger	1 sandwich	200
Chicken sandwich	1 sandwich	186
Fish sandwich	1 sandwich	155
French fries	1 order	301
Hamburger	1 sandwich	161
Onion chips	1 order	329
Onion rings	1 order	245
Sausage & egg sandwich	1 sandwich	322
Sausage sandwich	1 sandwich	196
WHITEFISH, LAKE:		
Baked, stuffed	4 oz.	244
Smoked	4 oz.	176
WIENER WRAP (Pillsbury)	1 piece	60
WILD BERRY DRINK,		
canned (Hi-C)	6 fl. oz.	92
WINCHELL'S DONUT HOUSE:		
Buttermilk, old fashioned	2-oz. piece	249
Cake, devil's food, iced	2-oz. piece	241
Cinnamon crumb	2-oz. piece	240
Iced, chocolate	2-oz. piece	227
Raised, glazed	1¾-oz. piece	212
WINE (See specific type, such as CHIANTI, SHERRY, etc.)		
WINE, COOKING (Holland House):		
Marsala	1 fl. oz.	9
Red	1 fl. oz.	6
Sherry	1 fl. oz.	5
Vermouth or white	1 fl. oz.	1

Food and Description	Measure or Quantity	Calories
WINE COOLER (Bartles & Jaymes):		
Light berry	6 fl. oz.	71
Premium berry, premium peach or premium red sangria	6 fl. oz.	107
Premium black cherry	6 fl. oz.	104
Premium original	6 fl. oz.	99

Y

Food and Description	Measure or Quantity	Calories
YEAST, BAKER'S (Fleischmann's):		
Dry, active	1 packet	20
Fresh & household, active	.6-oz. cake	15
YOGURT:		
Regular:		
Plain:		
(Dannon):		
Low-fat	8-oz. cont.	110
Non-fat	8-oz. cont.	140
(Friendship)	8-oz. container	150
(Johanna)	8-oz. container	150
Lite-Line (Borden)	8-oz. container	140
(Meadow Gold)	8-oz. container	160
(Whitney's)	6-oz. container	150
Yoplait, regular	6-oz. container	130
Apple (Dannon) dutch, Fruit-on-the-Bottom	8-oz. container	240
Apple & raisins (Whitney's)	6-oz. container	200
Banana:		
(Dannon) Fruit-on-the-Bottom	8-oz. container	240
Yoplait, regular	6-oz. container	190
Blueberry:		
(Breyer's)	8-oz. container	260
(Dannon) *Fresh Flavors*	8-oz. container	200
(Mountain High)	8-oz. container	220
(Sweet 'n Low)	8-oz. container	150
(Whitney's)	6-oz. container	200
Yoplait, custard style	6-oz. container	190
Boysenberry:		
(Dannon) Fruit-on-the-Bottom	8-oz. container	240
(Sweet'n Low)	8-oz. container	150
Cherry:		
(Breyer's) black	8-oz. container	270
(Dannon) Fruit-on-the-Bottom	8-oz. container	240
(Sweet 'n Low)	8-oz. container	150
(Whitney's)	6-oz. container	200

Food and Description	Measure or Quantity	Calories
Yoplait:		
Breakfast yogurt, with almonds	6-oz. container	200
Custard style	6-oz. container	180
Light	6-oz. container	90
Cherry-vanilla (Borden) *Lite-Line*	8-oz. container	240
Coffee:		
(Colombo; Dannon)	8-oz. container	200
(Friendship)	8-oz. container	210
(Johanna)	8-oz. container	220
Exotic fruit (Dannon) Fruit-on-the-Bottom	8-oz. container	240
Lemon:		
(Dannon) *Fresh Flavors*	8-oz. container	200
(Johanna)	8-oz.container	220
(Sweet'n Low)	8-oz. container	150
(Whitney's)	6-oz. container	200
Yoplait:		
Regular	6-oz. container	190
Custard style	6-oz. container	190
Mixed berries (Dannon):		
Extra Smooth	4.4-oz. container	130
Fruit-on-the-Bottom	8-oz. container	240
Orange, *Yoplait*	6-oz. container	190
Peach:		
(Breyer's)	8-oz. container	270
(Dannon) Fruit-on-the-Bottom	8-oz. container	240
(Friendship)	8-oz. container	240
Lite-Line (Borden)	8-oz. container	230
(Sweet'n Low)	8-oz. container	150
(Whitney's)	6-oz. container	200
Yoplait:		
Regular	6-oz. container	190
Light	6-oz. container	90
Piña colada:		
(Dannon) Fruit-on-the-Bottom	8-oz. container	240
(Friendship)	8-oz. container	230
Yoplait, custard style	6-oz. container	190
Pineapple:		
(Breyer's)	8-oz. container	270
(Light n' Lively)	8-oz. container	240
Yoplait	6-oz. container	190
Raspberry:		
(Breyer's) red	8-oz. container	260
(Dannon):		
Extra Smooth	4.4-oz. container	130
Fresh Flavors	8-oz. container	200
(Light n' Lively) red	8-oz. container	230

Food and Description	Measure or Quantity	Calories
(Sweet'n Low)	8-oz container	150
Yoplait:		
Regular	6-oz. container	190
Custard style	6-oz. container	190
Light container	6-oz.	90
Strawberry:		
(Breyer's)	8-oz. container	270
(Dannon) *Fresh Flavors*	8-oz. container	200
(Friendship)	8-oz. container	230
(Light n' Lively)	8-oz. container	240
Lite-Line (Borden)	8-oz. container	240
(Meadow Gold)	8-oz. container	270
(Whitney's)	6-oz. container	200
Yoplait, light	6-oz. container	90
Strawberry-banana (Light n' Lively)	8-oz. container	260
Vanilla:		
(Breyer's)	8-oz. container	230
(Dannon) light, regular or cherry	8-oz. container	100
(Friendship)	8-oz. container	210
Yoplait, custard style	6-oz. container	180
Frozen, hard:		
Banana, *Danny-in-a-Cup*	8-oz. cup	210
Boysenberry, *Danny-On-A-Stick,* carob coated	2½-fl.-oz. bar	140
Boysenberry swirl (Bison)	¼ of 16-oz. container	116
Chocolate:		
(Bison)	¼ of 16-oz. container	116
(Colombo) bar, chocolate coated	1 bar	145
(Dannon):		
Danny-in-a-Cup	8-fl.-oz. cup	190
Danny-On-A-Stick, chocolate coated	2½-fl.-oz. bar	130
Chocolate chip (Bison)	¼ of 16-oz. container	116
Chocolate chocolate chip (Colombo)	4-oz. serving	150
Mocha (Colombo) bar	1 bar	80
Piña colada:		
(Colombo)	4-oz. serving	110
(Dannon):		
(*Danny-in-a-Cup*	8-oz. cup	210
Danny-On-A-Stick	2½-fl.-oz. bar	65
Raspberry, red (Dannon):		
Danny-in-a-Cup	8-oz. container	210
Danny-On-A-Stick, chocolate coated	2½-fl.-oz. bar	130

Food and Description	Measure or Quantity	Calories
Strawberry:		
(Bison)	¼ of 16-oz. container	116
(Colombo):		
Regular	4-oz. serving	110
Bar	1 bar	80
(Dannon):		
Danny-in-a-Cup	8 fl. oz.	210
Danny-Yo	3½ fl. oz.	110
Vanilla:		
(Colombo):		
Regular	4-oz. serving	110
Bar, chocolate coated	1 bar	145
(Dannon):		
Danny-in-a-Cup	8 fl. oz.	180
Danny-On-A-Stick	2½-fl.-oz. bar	65
Danny-Yo	3½-oz. serving	110
Frozen, soft (Colombo)	6-fl.-oz. serving	130
YOGURT BAR, frozen (Dole):		
Cherry	1 bar	80
Chocolate or strawberry	1 bar	70
Strawberry-banana	1 bar	60

Z

Food and Description	Measure or Quantity	Calories
ZINFANDEL WINE (Louis M. Martini) regular vintage	3 fl. oz.	64
ZINGERS (Dolly Madison):		
Devils food	1¼-oz. piece	140
Raspberry	1¼-oz. piece	130
ZWEIBACK (Gerber; Nabisco)	1 piece	30